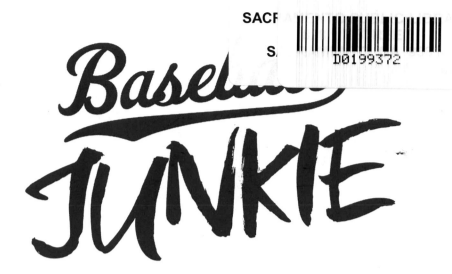

Baseball JUNKIE

THE RISE, FALL AND REDEMPTION OF A WORLD SERIES CHAMPION

AUBREY HUFF
STEPHEN CASSAR

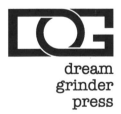

dream
grinder
press

SAN DIEGO, CALIFORNIA

DreamGrinder Press, Inc.
San Diego, California
www.dreamgrinderpress.com

Publisher's Cataloging-in-Publication data

Names: Huff, Aubrey, author. | Cassar, Stephen, author.

Title: Baseball junkie : the rise , fall , and redemption of a World Series champion / Aubrey Huff; with Stephen Cassar.
Description: San Diego, CA: DreamGrinder Press, 2017.
Identifiers: ISBN 978-0-9984407-0-5
Subjects: LCSH Huff, Aubrey. | Baseball players--United States--Biography. | Recovering addicts--United States--Biography. | BISAC BIOGRAPHY & AUTOBIOGRAPHY / Sports

Classification: LCC GV865 .H84 H84 2017| DDC 796.357092--dc23

Publisher's Note: Some names and identifying details have been changed to protect the privacy of individuals.

Edited by Susan Ray and Carlos de los Rios.
Cover design by Greg Jackson, ThinkPen Design.
Author photo (c) 2016 Deborah Cartwright, Del Mar Photographics.
Interior design and layout by Stephen Cassar.

Typeset in Rosarivo 10pt. Copyright (c) 2012 Pablo Ugerman, and Hattori Hanzo 14pt. Copyright (c) 2010 Roman Shamin

Contact DreamGrinder Press for quantity discounts.

Baseball Junkie/ Aubrey Huff. -- 1st ed.
ISBN 978-0-9984407-0-5

ver. 3 - 01/11/17

For my wife Baubi.

I can't even imagine where I would be today without you in my life.
You have one of the strongest, most loving, passionate,
and forgiving hearts I've ever known.

I'm so thankful God gave me you.
You have turned me into the man I'm proud to be today.
Thank you so much for standing beside me in the midst of my
unending faults and struggles. How you're still with me is
a miracle from God himself.

I love you,
Aubrey

INTRODUCTION

Game 4. October 28th. 2012 World Series. Detroit, Michigan. 42,152 screaming Tigers fans in attendance.

The cold breeze rips through the dugout as I sit bundled up in my thick Giants jacket. A space heater blows hot air two feet away from my face, but it's no match for the brisk Michigan night. I watch the action on the field, casually leaning up against the dugout netting. Miguel Cabrera, that year's Triple Crown winner strolls to the plate to face Sergio Romo. One out stands between us and our second World Series championship. The dugout sits on pins and needles, anxiously waiting, ready to charge the field to celebrate. We are just one pitch away from immortality. My mind races, fantasizing about the million places I would rather be. I hate baseball!

This book wasn't easy to write. As a matter of fact, it was one of the hardest things I have ever attempted, forcing me to take a long, hard look in the mirror and uncomfortably bare my soul to finish it. So why did I write it?

Four years have passed since my retirement. Four long years to contemplate my career and my life. I realized during that time that I have a story to tell and that maybe, just maybe, that story may inspire someone, give them hope. Yes, this book is about baseball, but it's also about my struggles and triumphs spanning a thirteen-year Major League Baseball career.

I was a desperate soul that let addiction, depression, anxiety, pride, fear, worry, selfishness, doubt, and a laundry list of other deadly sins cripple me to the point of suicidal thoughts for the majority of my life. If just one person reads this book and realizes they are not alone in their struggles, and maybe feels encouraged, then the pain of baring my soul is worth it. I have experienced a lot of pain in the last five years, pain I would not wish upon my worst enemy. But that doesn't even compare to the pain I caused the ones I love the most.

One book is not enough to tell you about all my degeneracy. I was an absolute scumbag most of my life, only interested in how I could benefit from someone else. I was a taker, not a giver. It was my way or the highway. I'm sorry to all the people who politely asked me for my autograph over the years only to have me sarcastically shun them. I'm sorry to the women I intentionally took advantage of in my younger days. I'm sorry to my ex-teammates and coaches for the train wreck you had to watch day in and day out. And most importantly, I'm sorry to my wife, Baubi, for the living hell I put her through all those years. Baubi, God certainly put you in my life to make me a better man. You have inspired me to become the man I am today, and for you, I am eternally grateful.

Friends, family, and teammates are probably going to think that there is no way I wrote this book. Many of you already know I may be street-smart, but book smart? Absolutely not!

Back as a teenager when I was looking at colleges to apply to, I, like millions of others before me, took the SAT, a test that most colleges use in determining admission. I remember that Saturday morning like it were yesterday. It was misting on my way to the Fort Worth Library, and underneath the Dallas Cowboys jacket I had on, I could feel sweat oozing out of my pores. I felt pretty nervous walking into that building, but as I sat working away on the three sections of the test with my number two pencil, something happened. I knew I wouldn't score a perfect 800 in each of the three sections, but I felt like I was truly acing it. The questions seemed almost too easy, like they were designed for a fourth-grader. I walked out of that library feeling pretty proud of myself, knowing I did well, firmly believing I could apply to almost any college I was interested in.

The letter delivered by the mailman six weeks later told a different story. My dear mom anxiously opened the envelope, and with a confused look on her face said to me, "Congratulations! You made a 600!"

Still convinced I had rocked that test, I asked: "Great! 600 for which part?"

She quickly replied, "No. 600 for the whole thing, Aubrey!"

Now keep in mind that back then you got 400 points just for writing your name on the top of the test papers!

I hope that as you read about my struggles and missteps, you will see that unless you have your eyes set on the right things in life, none of what you achieve or earn matters. The money, the fame, the material possessions, none of it.

I, Aubrey Lewis Huff III, have reached the pinnacle of Major League Baseball. I have won two World Series Championships with the San Francisco Giants. I have earned a lot of money playing baseball, and was fortunate enough to retire at the age of 36. I live in a beautiful home in Del Mar, California. I'm married to a smoking hot, supportive wife who I would give my life for, and I am a proud father to two healthy, happy, perfect little boys. I have a life that 99.9 percent of men in the world would absolutely kill for!

So how does a man who seemingly has everything by society's standards find himself suicidal in his closet one evening?

How does a "successful" man reach the conclusion that maybe the best thing to do is to finally end it all?

It's been four years since I picked up a bat, and I have to say that the years since have been the most challenging of my life. I've gone from the exciting fast-paced, well-traveled, adrenaline-fueled life of a professional athlete to a stay-at-home dad, relegated to folding laundry, doing dishes, grocery shopping, and cooking dinner. I oftentimes feel like a caged, castrated lion.

The addictive roar of 40,000-plus fans has been replaced with a deafening silence. The brotherhood and daily camaraderie of the locker room is long gone. I sometimes feel like the game, and even my old teammates, have forgotten about me. The confidence I used to have is fragile. I have struggled to find relevance in my life again.

That dreaded word "retirement" and the eerily quiet life that follows terrifies most professional athletes, but it is something I secretly wished for on many a six-hour plane flight during my career. But no amount of wishing or dreaming could have prepared me for the challenges waiting for me at the end of my career.

It felt great to finally finish this book. It took a year, but I feel like I finally got all the important parts of my journey so far down on paper. In many ways this process was very therapeutic, way cheaper than any shrink. The ups, the many downs, the disappointments and triumphs. I certainly had my doubts during the whole writing process with a tiny voice constantly whispering in my ears, *Your story sucks, Aubrey! It is not interesting. Nobody cares about a mediocre baseball player who has been out of the game for four years.* I think you will feel some of my pain and cringe at some of the stories in here. I won't ruin the ending for you, just know that there *is* hope.

Since my retirement, I have had to swallow my pride and accept who I have become as a man. Mentally, physically, emotionally, and most importantly, spiritually. I feel like I have finally found a huge light at the end of a long, dark tunnel.

My friends, I have learned we all have our struggles. Chances are you'll identify with some of mine. If so, my hope is that you will be encouraged. It's never too late to make a change. You may not believe what I believe, or agree with everything in here. I don't want you to think for a second that I'm on my high horse preaching to you, but please keep an open mind and a soft heart as you dive into my journey. I look back at those difficult moments since retirement now, and am so thankful that I went through them. I knew back then that I needed a massive change in my life, but change for the better never comes easy.

I have changed, but don't get me wrong, I am no saint. I still curse like I'm in a major league dugout. I still have a few too many on occasion. And my wife will tell you that I still complain, a lot! But I can truly say that I'm a different person today than those that know me remember. I'm a better husband, father, and friend. I'm a better man. And I know for a fact that I could never have done it on my own.

CHAPTER ONE
ATTACK IN NEW YORK

*"Money can't buy you happiness,
but it does bring you a more
pleasant form of misery."*

—SPIKE MILLIGAN

April 21st, 2012: New York City as a San Francisco Giant.

I remember that night like it was yesterday. I remember the exact time my life began to unravel, pushing me down a path that would change my life forever.

It was a Saturday day game against the Mets and it was a grind from the get-go. Our whole team seemed flat for the first eight innings, lacking any fire or enthusiasm. We were losing the game 4-1 headed into the top of the ninth.

I stood at first base the entire game, uninterested, unengaged. I was there in body, but my mind drifted. All I could think about was how much I missed my wife, Baubi, and the kids back in Tampa; and how the game of baseball was sucking the life out of me. I was off to one of the worst starts of my career offensively, hitting .188. For a guy making $10 million a year, that was an absolute disgrace. But the real disgrace was that I really didn't give a damn.

Baseball was all I knew and believed in. It was all I lived and breathed since I was old enough to swing a bat. Other than my family, it was all I had ever truly loved. Now all I had to look forward to after that game was another miserable night's sleep in another lonely hotel room 1100 miles from home.

Major League Baseball is hands-down the best job in the world when you are young and single. You get to travel to bustling big cities and live in an unreal parallel universe in the spotlight of the media and adoration of fans. But when you have a wife and children, the loneliness of the road gets to you.

The travel schedule is brutal, putting you on the road for weeks on end. Not getting a chance to kiss your wife goodnight, or tuck your kids in night after night really gets to you. The media attention you once sought becomes your relentless enemy, watching for chinks in your armor. Chinks that members of the media pick at until they get the story they need.

Here I was in one of the world's greatest cities having just played a nail-biter against the New York Mets. I should have been thrilled to be knee-deep in a pro ball career, playing on one of the world's biggest stages. I had everything I had ever dreamed of, including a beautiful wife, two healthy, happy, handsome boys, and a salary most men can only dream about. I had succeeded on every level measurable by any American standard. And I hated everything and everybody, including myself.

The very thing that I had worked so hard for since I was 10 years old, my dream, was becoming my worst nightmare. I despised the game of baseball. It had become my prison.

The loneliness, almost unbearable pressure, and performance anxiety that continues to build at this level of the game ensures that no amount of money can put a smile on your face. The simple game I grew up loving was now just a job. I was just punching the clock like my old man before me in his dead-end electrician job.

I know what you're thinking right about now. *Here is this dude making a truckload of money playing America's favorite pastime, and he's complaining? What the hell is wrong with him? After all, it's not even real work! It's just a game!* Believe me, I agree. I have been to a lot of shrinks to help me figure that one out!

So as you can tell by now, I was having a real tough time finding excitement and joy in the game. To make matters worse, it was just the first month of a long season, and I already had a countdown calendar hanging on the wall. Each day I would check off a square, like a kid waiting anxiously for Christmas.

Top of the ninth inning. I slumped back against the dugout wall and fiddled with my batting gloves. We needed a big rally to get back into this game and I was hitting second. I dragged my bat up the steps onto the on deck circle pretending I cared as I swung my bat for show. I jealously eyed Buster Posey stride to the plate. He had that look in his eyes. The look that I used to have when I was that young into my career. The kid bounced on the first pitch and led us off with a solid single up the middle. Nice start to the inning.

I can't say I felt confident taking my turn at bat. I had been the rally killer so often this first month that I couldn't even look up as I lugged my six-foot-four-inch frame to the plate, eyes transfixed on the ground, the bat feeling like it weighed 100 pounds. I halfheartedly dug into the batter's box in time for the windup. I grounded the first pitch weakly back to the pitcher and began the embarrassing jog to first hoping the pitcher wouldn't throw the ball away so I could crawl back to the dugout and sulk. My wish was granted as the out was recorded effortlessly. I remember thinking on the slow jog back to the dugout that even a kid could have hit the ball further.

With me out of the way at least the guys now had a chance to mount a comeback as the next few batters began to show signs of life. We scored a run. 4-2. I could have cared less as I warmed the bench. I was too busy looking down with dejection, hoping we didn't tie this thing up and go into extra innings!

I was off daydreaming about something when our manager Bruce Bochy walked up to me. "You ever played second base, son?" I wasn't sure what to say. Of course not! Second base was reserved for players who were good defenders, and those words were never ones I'd heard any coach utter about me. I was mostly a first baseman much of my life and had never played second, not even in tee-ball.

Bruce didn't wait for an answer. He took one look and knew what I was thinking. He looked me square in the eyes and spoke clearly and slowly with a serious look on his face. "Sorry, Huffy. If they score next inning and tie the game up, I have no other option but to put you in at second. We're out of infielders." I nodded an "okay," not panicking too much about it. After all, we still needed to score two more runs with two outs.

To my horror, I watched Nate Schierholtz walk, then Emmanuel Burris get a single. The game had suddenly returned from beyond the grave.

Pinch hitter Brandon Belt was sent to the plate with a simple mission: drive one into the gap. Bring the guys home. He hit a towering fly ball to shallow center field. An easy play that should have sealed the victory for the Mets. But this was no ordinary day in Flushing Meadows. Wind gusts were whipping through the stadium making any pop-up less than routine. Belt's pop-up twisted in the wind and landed untouched in shallow center field scoring two runs. 4-4. The crowd was on the edge of their seats now and fans that were halfway out the stadium trying to beat the mad rush, turned back, grabbing the first available open seat to see how this thing was going to end.

I am not sure what happened next on the field because I was too busy rummaging around the dugout, asking around and desperately trying on infield gloves to find one that felt okay. I didn't own a middle infielders glove. All I had was my first baseman's mitt and an outfielder's glove. And those wouldn't do.

Angel Pagan struck out for out number three. Here we go. Bottom of the ninth. It was time to make my debut at second base at Citi Field in front of 33,844 in attendance! I settled in at second, secretly hoping they wouldn't hit it to me. And if you know the game of baseball, you know that Murphy's Law applies in spades in this game. Just thinking it pretty much guaranteed I was going to get a ball hit directly at me. A little voice in my head taunted me, *The ball will always find you, Huffy! Always.*

Okay. I've got this, I reassured myself. Mets first baseman Lucas Duda led off with a single. The little kid in me got excited for a minute. *It would be so badass if I had a chance to turn a double play!* I could see it clearly in my mind's eye. I saw myself making the play of the game, making ESPN Sports Center's top 10 plays. It would be a top 10 play all right, just the not-so-top 10 plays. Like a kid at practice, anticipating the ball, I got ready. I could already hear the applause. My mind played the slow-motion replay. I could hear the roar of the Giants fans who had made it out to Citi Field that sunny Saturday afternoon rose to a crescendo, no doubt very impressed with my smooth moves.

The very next batter was Mets catcher Josh Thole. He hit a sharp ground ball straight to our shortstop Manny Burriss. My cue. Time to spring into action.

In professional baseball you have to possess killer instincts. I had fine-tuned mine over 15 years of pro ball conditioning, and they kicked in now. Except instead of breaking to second to take the throw from Manny to start the double play, I instinctively broke to first base to receive the throw, just like I had done countless other times in my career.

Manny pumped-faked a throw to second, fully expecting someone (me) to be there, and of course nobody was, because I was on my way to first base. I'd just killed us. My hesitation cost us the game. Not only was the runner safe at second, but now we had a player on first to contend with. I felt like an idiot and could just hear the air get sucked out of our dugout and the hordes of Giants fans in the stands. What should have been a routine play let the Mets get the upper hand in a game that had no margin for error. And we were about to pay the price.

Walk. Infield single. Bases were loaded now with one out. Mets center fielder Kirk Nieuwenhuis stepped to the plate with the game on the line. I was begging for Kirk to end the game so I could retreat to the locker room in my shame. Brandon Belt had replaced me defensively at first base when he pinch hit, and Nieuwenhuis hit a sharp ground ball directly to him.

There was only one play here. We couldn't let the runner from third score. Brandon tossed the ball home for out number two. Buster Posey sprang into action going for the third out. He now had a moving target in pitcher Jeremy Affelt covering first base, but his throw sailed high down the right field line. And just like that, the game was over. The runner from second rounded third, scoring easily. Game over! And the start of the bottom of the ninth inning of my career.

The next 48 hours were a blur.

After the game, the media, of course, blamed me for the blunder. I was guilty for not doing my job and breaking to second. It was an honest mistake, but I knew I had screwed up. I had let my team down. As I look back, one thing in my career I can say I am proud of is that no matter how embarrassing or how stupid my errors, I always took responsibility. So I took the heat, and owned my mistake.

So right about now you may be thinking, *Here we go. I see where this is going. Just another poor ex-pro athlete looking for sympathy from the outside world because he couldn't hack it under pressure, even when he was making guaranteed millions. If only he knew what REAL work was!* The fact was, however, that I wasn't mentally *in* that game. I had checked out long before that, way back at the beginning of the season.

I let our loyal fans and teammates down that night because I was just going through the motions. And baseball demands— no, deserves—more than that. Baseball expects discipline, passion, and precision. My focus on the field had to be laser-sharp. My mind had to be fully in the game with no reservations. Every single day. Every single play. Anything less was unacceptable; I knew this. But my brain was foggy that day, even catatonic. Our fans, my teammates, and our coaches deserved my best and I was at a point in my career where I couldn't give it to them.

I was playing naked that game. Like a nightmare that I still suffer from today. This was the first season since 2008 that I had played without at least 20 milligrams of Adderall coursing through my veins. I had quit it cold turkey in an attempt to get back what this prescription drug had taken away. I knew I had to push on and get my life back, but nothing could have prepared me for what it felt like to play without it. There is no other way to describe it. Naked was exactly what I felt like for the entire first month of that season.

At the end of the game, I didn't feel like heading back to the hotel room. I needed to forget. I agreed to dinner plans with some of my friends and family—my half-brother Chris Dickerson; Brett Pill, a backup first baseman on the Giants; and Justin Turner, utility infielder for the Mets.

I don't remember the name of the restaurant where we ate, or what I ordered. I was more focused on my liquid intake, flowing through my usual six to 10 beers during the course of dinner. *Gotta get numb, and go get 'em tomorrow.* The night was young, so Brian Packin, a good friend of mine who lived in the city, got us all into a popular hangout.

At this lounge, I squirmed in my seat as the replay of my mental miscue appeared on the television above the bar. Here I was trying to escape the game, drowning my worries away; and everywhere I went, there it was for the entire world to see!

It wasn't that the play bothered me all that much. After all, it was my first appearance at second base, ever. It was just an honest mistake. But I felt like the weight of the world had just settled on my shoulders, and the gaze of hundreds of thousands of disappointed fans was boring into the back of my skull as I sat there. I had never felt this sad, angry, disappointed, ashamed, and numb before. I remember thinking as I took a sip of my beer how much I hated playing major league baseball, and how I wished I could just go back home to Tampa right then and there. *Screw the fame, the money, the fans, my teammates!*

Be careful what you wish for, my friends!

When I finally stumbled back into my hotel room around one a.m., I fell right into the bed. I was too drunk to feel sorry for myself. I didn't even take off my clothes that night. I remember feeling the mattress push back against my full weight, and the bed rock back and forth a little, almost like it was a waterbed, or as if I was laying in the hull of a small sailboat. I dangled one foot off the side. *Ahhh... I can finally close my eyes and forget about life for a bit.*

I woke suddenly. The bright red numbers on the alarm clock burned into the back of my eyes. It said it was three a.m. I stumbled toward the bathroom, desperately searching the wall for a light switch. I remember taking a leak for what seemed like minutes, with the room spinning around me, and the porcelain bowl coming closer and then moving farther away as I stood with both feet firmly planted, trying to stabilize the room as I swayed like a ship in a storm. It was a feeling I had known almost nightly since I was in college.

Stumbling back to my bed, a sudden chill ran through my veins, starting in my chest and quickly making it all the way through my entire body. The walls of my room were closing in on me. My heart started to race like I had never felt it race before. My breathing became so shallow that I thought I was going to hyperventilate. As if in a dream, I struggled to put one foot in front of the other, like a guy taking a sobriety test after a cop pulls him over. I felt alone and terrified. I was confused and disoriented. I was convinced I was about to drop dead.

I made it to the window and yanked the curtains open with one fluid motion. I fumbled with the window handle for a few seconds and got the window partially open, just enough to steal a lungful of polluted New York air. The big bright lights of the "city that never sleeps" seemed surreal. They felt like bright laser beams as they hit the back my retina. I felt a sharp pain in my head from the early stages of a hangover. City that never sleeps? I felt like I was about to take a permanent sleep!

All of a sudden I wasn't drunk anymore. Adrenaline kicked in and my brain switched to survival mode.

I turned from the window and took a deep breath. *I'm having a heart attack.* My heart was trying to punch its way out of my chest cavity. My head felt like a horse had just kicked me square in the teeth. I had been smashed in the left temple before, when I got hit by a baseball in 2000. The surgeon told me back then that if the orbital fracture was just a millimeter longer, I would have lost sight in that eye. To say that having your eyeball dangle there just barely in its socket was painful, would be a gross understatement. I walk around today with two screws around my left eye because of that. Yes, that injury sucked. But this felt worse. I had never experienced a state of panic like this.

As a player you learn to deal with the cruelest mind games courtesy of your opponent, but mostly yourself. The late Yogi Berra said it best: "90 percent of the game is half mental." In baseball, you learn to deal with fear and frustration because that's the world you live in day in, day out. You learn that the best way to keep things in check is to bottle it all up, and pop an Adderall. At least that's how I chose to deal with it. Your mind is quite literally the biggest thing you need a handle on in order to be a successful baseball player, but now I felt like I was losing it. Instinct kicked in. I frantically shoved my clothes and belongings in my bag. I had to get the hell out of Dodge. I remember thinking, *I'm not dying here in this hotel room. I have to get home to my wife and kids. I have to say good-bye before I die!*

So, drenched in a nervous sweat and still wearing the clothes from the night before, I dragged my bag behind me down to the lobby. Not sure how, but apparently I hopped in a cab.

The next thing I knew I was standing in front of an American Airlines counter at JFK Airport. I know I looked like death and smelled worse, with booze oozing out of every pore on my body. I looked drunk, but worse still, also like I'd just been in a bout with Mike Tyson. Strangely, I felt sober as a judge.

"Son, are you okay?" the lady behind the counter asked. I am sure that the way I looked, smelled, and slurred my speech was raising all kinds of red flags. I muttered, "I'm just really hungover, and want to get home." She quickly booked me on the next flight.

That hour-long wait at the gate seemed like days. I sprawled out on the floor, staring at the airport ceiling with my feet propped up against the wall. Beads of sweat ran down my forehead, dripping into my ear canals. The firm, cold tile floor felt good against my back, offering relief for my hot skin.

Finally, time to board. I shuffled anxiously onto the plane, trying to keep my distance from those around me. I sank into my window seat in coach. The strangest mix of emotions crept into my brain as I buckled in and reason slowly returned. Part of me was happy that I would finally see my family after two weeks on the road. The other part of me was devastated by the previous night's game. My heart was still pounding, head throbbing. I couldn't believe how all rationale seemed to have fallen out of my 20th-story hotel window that night. Baseball had been the last thing on my mind. Survival was the only option. I knew I had to get home to Baubi and the kids, but I couldn't believe I was ready to so easily abandon my teammates and coaches, people who really cared for me.

Then came confusion. What had just happened a few hours ago in the hotel room? Had I suffered a stroke? A mild heart attack? What the hell was going on with me?

As I was busy contemplating life, seemingly out of nowhere, the plane door slammed shut. That loud bang felt almost like a bomb, the percussion from the blast pounding my chest. I was back in overdrive. A voice came over the PA system, something about *all electronics off.*

This feeling was new. I had never been claustrophobic or scared to fly, but as the door slammed shut, the cabin contracted around me. The whole plane seemed to be getting shorter, just like my breathing. Part of me wanted to scream to the flight attendant that I wanted to get off. But I knew I couldn't do that. I knew I had to get the hell out of New York City. I had to see my family again.

As my heart pumped 200 beats a minute, I am sure I had a look on my face like a caged animal's, so I was glad nobody was sitting next to me. I was still sweating profusely and now began shaking head to toe. I reached up for the air vents above, but had to close my eyes. I felt around till I found the little knob jutting out of them and aimed the little cold air streams straight at my face. *I can breathe.* I applied my mental conditioning in a desperate attempt to lower my heart rate. It didn't really work, but I managed to talk myself off the ledge just enough to maybe survive the flight.

The thrust of the jets pushed me back into the seat, as I clenched my hands together and closed my eyes. I prayed the entire flight home, begging God to forgive me for a life lived selfishly. I pleaded to him for another chance. To not die here alone on this cold empty plane. Tears began dripping down my face as I pondered the constant sin of my major league baseball career. I felt every emotion under the sun, again moving from guilt, to rage, to disappointment and sadness. I prayed harder. For peace. For forgiveness.

That two-and-a-half-hour flight felt a lot longer. I sat frozen in my seat the whole time, too afraid to get up. I needed to take a leak so bad I could taste it, but I held it. I stared at the back of the seat in front of me. Too embarrassed to look around and make eye contact with anyone.

Then the weirdest thing happened. As soon as the captain's voice trailed off over the intercom: "Ladies and gentlemen, we are about 15 minutes out of Tampa. Please return to your seats, fasten your seat belts, return tray tables to their full upright position, sit back, relax, and enjoy the rest of your flight," a sense of calm washed over me. He said *relax*, and my mind listened!

I raised the sunshade and glanced out the window to my left. The sun was rising over the familiar downtown Tampa skyline. My heart rate slowed. My mind came back into focus. *I'm not going to die.*

Again, I questioned my sanity. *What the hell was that all about? What now? Do I go straight to a hospital? What do I tell Baubi? She thinks I am still in New York!*

The tires met the runway with a squeal and a puff of smoke. I inhaled a lungful of stale airplane air, and with it, relief. I was home!

CHAPTER TWO
PRAYING FOR RAIN

*"Happiness is waking up
without a hangover."*

–ROBERT BLACK

July 18th, 2009: Chicago

Saturday morning. Chicago White Sox visiting clubhouse as a Baltimore Oriole.

Ask any pro, and they'll tell you the same thing. Regardless of how well any season starts, or how pure your intentions, losing game after game starts to drag you down. You soon find yourself not really firing on all cylinders. Going through the motions. And we were halfway through a really putrid season.

It was the second game of a three-game weekend series. The White Sox had beaten us Friday night 12-8. Like many of my teammates, I was abusing my body on a daily basis, on and off the field. The aches, pains, and mental grind of the game were starting to mount. And here I was back for another ass kicking.

I sought out a dark, secret part of the facility that was off-limits to the media. Every clubhouse seemed to have at least one of these secret corners, and I loved them. They felt like the only place I could be alone with my thoughts...and hangovers. I sank into an old, smelly, black La-Z-Boy with no intention of getting up anytime soon. I could smell years of sweat and history in that clubhouse.

It was a one p.m. day game. Again, here I was miles away from home, feeling the full weight of the booze from the night before, and in absolutely no mood to suit up or play ball. I closed my eyes for a few minutes and played through the years and years spent on losing teams, getting my teeth kicked in on a daily basis, suffering under the weight of the never-ending grind of the game.

I buried my face in my hands for a minute trying to massage the deep throbbing pain that was just an inch out of reach beneath my temples. It would be another eight days before I got to see Baubi and my handsome one-year-old boy Jayce. But before I flew home to Baltimore for the next home stand, we'd have to face the American League East powerhouses, the New York Yankees and the Boston Red Sox, on their own turf.

Someone once said, "It's not whether you win or lose, it's how you play the game." Well, that someone obviously never played professional sports. Losing sucks. I knew. Six seasons dead last in Tampa, and now deep into the second straight losing season in Baltimore. I would have killed to be in the thick of a playoff drive.

It's funny that as a kid, all I could think about was getting to the big leagues. Making it. Yet as a pro, all I could now think about was getting back to that feeling of when I was a little leaguer... when the game was so new and exciting, I could hardly contain my emotions. But try as I might to bring back that passion, I just couldn't. Here I was in my early 30s when I should really have been hitting my stride, and I was completely over it.

At this point, I was getting used to losing. I was to be a free agent in the coming offseason, and the years of abuse were showing in my swing and performance. I had dug myself into a pretty deep hole statistically. I just knew we were going to get swept by the White Sox before our trip to New York, but I had to get out there and play well the rest of the year, or face the reality of a life without baseball.

The Orioles were paying me regardless of how I played. I was on the last year of a $20-million, three-year deal, and my commitment to the team was marginal at best. To put it bluntly, most days I felt like I was wearing a black ski mask, stealing money. My take for a few hours on the field that afternoon would net me over $41,000, roughly what my dad made breaking his back in a whole year. And I didn't appreciate it. Quite frankly, even at a million dollars a game, I still would not have enjoyed it.

I sat there nursing a nice fizzy Alka-Seltzer Morning Relief, my "coffee" of choice on days like this. I dozed in and out of sleep. Every few minutes, my gut contracted and bubbled. I could taste vomit in my mouth.

It was pushing 11:30, and here I was in sliding shorts, T-shirt, and shower shoes, still wearing a five-o'clock shadow from the night before, feeling, looking, and smelling like absolute death.

I heard someone walk in. I looked up with one eye half open. Here was a teammate, fully suited in spikes, ready to play. I will call him 'Ryan'. He was staring right at me with a smirk on his face.

"Tough one last night, Huffy?" he asked with a laugh. That was an understatement! At that moment, I would rather have been anywhere instead of having to face tens of thousands of Chicago fans.

"I've got something that will make you feel invincible." I perked up, both eyes open now. Realizing he had my attention, Ryan continued, "Have you ever been popped for failing a drug test?"

In Major League Baseball, players would be drug-tested randomly when we least expected it, and at that time, if you failed a drug test for any performance enhancing drug, you simply got away with a slap on the wrist. Nobody knew about it but you and the players' union. However, if you got caught a second time, things got serious. It would cost you a suspension of up to 50 games with no pay. A third offense, and you would be kissing your career good-bye.

"No. Never been popped," I replied, still intrigued by this magic "invincibility" concoction. "What you got?"

Ryan launched into a quick intro to Adderall that may as well have been a radio ad for the drug. It sounded amazing and harmless. Apparently, this was a drug they prescribed to kids for attention deficit hyperactivity disorder. How bad could it be? He told me all I had to do was take one pill and wait thirty minutes for it to kick in. I was sold. A few seconds later, a shiny capsule filled with hope and promise sat in my hand, looking back at me with its white top, orange bottom, and black lettering. It looked like a miniature Oriole dressed and ready for action in his Friday orange uniform.

I sank back in the recliner eyeing it, not even realizing that Ryan had left the room. The pill seemed small in my hand, so light. Almost like it was hollow.

I won't feel anything from this thing, I thought. *And I couldn't possibly feel any worse than I do right now. Screw it!*

I chased it with a swig of water and swallowed. As it slid down my throat I felt the smooth edges force their way down my throat, quickly followed by an instant jolt of regret. *What have*

I just ingested? What have I done? Part of me wanted to go to the bathroom, shove my fingers down my throat, and get it back out of me. But I simply sat there instead, alone in the darkened room waiting for the invincible feeling I was promised.

Up to this point, drugs of any kind scared me to death. Other than the occasional Advil, I avoided foreign substances like the plague. In fact, the only time I had ever done any drugs in my life was during my college days where I got into the social weed scene. But even then, weed was never something I ever felt I absolutely needed, or got addicted to. I just smoked weed to fit in. To help me feel like part of the group. But I had hated it. Smoking made me feel depressed, and took away my motivation and drive. I felt like a zombie on marijuana. I promised myself then I'd never take another drug in my life. Yet, here I now was, breaking my own promise, popping a chemical into my body I knew absolutely nothing about.

10 minutes passed. It was almost noon. Quite literally out of nowhere, the dim lights of the room began to get brighter. It was like someone had walked up to the light switch and turned one of those old dimmer knobs (like those in every American dining room) all the way to high. Except it looked brighter than that. It seemed almost like someone had just traded the dim incandescent bulbs for those fancy halogen types. I now could see every nook and cranny of the room I was in. The dark corners were no longer dark. I could see every mark and stain on the carpet. Every scratch on the wall. Every imperfection on the ceiling. My first instinct was that there had to be some problem with the electrical system in the building. The lights were bright, but it wasn't like staring at the sun. The light had a weird aura about it. Crisp. Clean. Clear.

The air began to smell cleaner in that damp back room. It felt almost like someone had magically sucked out 18 years of musty, mildewy air, and replaced it with crisp, mountain air. Like a fresh breeze captured right after a snowfall high up at a ski resort and magically transported to the U.S. Cellular Field visiting clubhouse.

The pounding in my head and the intense pressure on my temples disappeared as quickly as they had come on.

Wow!

I sprang out of the chair and hustled over to the locker room, looking for my savior's locker. I felt a surge of excitement. "Thanks, man. This stuff is amazing!" I said with a newfound spark in my eyes. I had never felt this alive! Or *this* ready to play the game. He just gave me a proud knowing smile.

I was so excited to get out on the field; I couldn't get my jersey and spikes on fast enough.

I have always been the kind of guy who hated going out early onto the field. I just dreaded emerging out of the tunnel to be greeted by thousands of annoying fans. Most days, I was the last guy walking out to stretch. But here I was, 45 minutes until game time, ready for action! I beat our strength coach out to the right field line to stretch. As a matter of fact, I was the first player on either team to take the field that day to get loose, even beating both starting pitchers out there!

Stepping out of that tunnel felt like I was just coming out of my mother's womb as a baby. The minute I stepped out into the stadium, I marveled at everything around me. I noticed so many things I hadn't noticed in a long, long time. The blue sky was simply magnificent; the smell of the freshly cut, bright green grass was sensory overload.

Sounds were crisp and pleasant. It felt like someone had just turned the volume up on the sounds I loved, and way down on the sounds I hated.

I remember lying face down on the grass down the right field line getting ready to stretch. Breathing it in for what seemed like minutes. Yes, I was breathing in the grass! It no doubt must have looked like I had lost my marbles. But I didn't give a damn. I was totally lost and free in the moment. Not even the heckling Chicago fans bothered me!

Now I don't want to glorify a drug that has caused so much destruction in my life, but Ryan was right. Adderall truly made me feel invincible. One pill and I was simply oblivious to any negative feeling, any sense of doubt, worry, misery, or fear. Life was never more beautiful. The performance anxiety that I was so used to feeling before each game was completely gone. Just like that! I felt a feeling of euphoria coursing through my brain. *How in the hell have I ever played baseball without this stuff?*

Performance-wise, my first game on the drug was no different than most games that season. I finished that game 0-for-4 with a strikeout. What *had* changed however, was my attitude. It was the most fun I had ever had playing in the big leagues. I felt like a superhero on deck, even though the results told a different story. Nothing scared me. Nothing could hurt me.

As a team, we were trailing the Sox by a run late in the game. I was the designated hitter for the day, and as I leaned over the dugout railings, enjoying the best seat in the house, I found myself praying we would score just one more run to tie the game and go to extra innings. I desperately wanted to keep playing.

That was certainly a first for me. Usually by the third inning I would be begging for the game to be over, or a storm to blow in and rain us out, anything to end the misery. But I was completely in the moment with tons of energy. With the Adderall, the aching body from the dog days of summer was gone, and I morphed from the quiet guy on the team to the Vince Lombardi of the Orioles.

Here I was, cheering my team on like a softball girl from the top railing of the dugout. I felt like a kid playing baseball again. No pressure. Just a pure love for the beautiful game.

I'm never playing another game without this stuff! I was hooked.

I now realize why drug pushers hang around schools giving away free samples. I needed more of this stuff before the next game. Only problem was, how was I going to get a therapeutic use exemption from the league at my age? Adderall is commonly prescribed for people with ADHD. Here I was at 33, and I somehow suddenly developed ADHD? Likely story!

I had to go back to the source. He had to know how to get the exemption I needed. I had to get one to make sure that if I ever got popped, the league had documentation and could explain why I tested positive for the speed (because that's basically what Adderall is).

While I was shopping this book around looking for an agent to help me get it published, I was told I should name names, exposing the Adderall racket inside the league for what it is. I was told to specifically name the teammate who gave me my first pill, and to rat out everyone else that was involved. I was told outright that unless I did this, basically threw friends, teammates and colleagues under the bus, my book would be boring and would certainly not be a success. I have to say I was blown away by that. Did I really have to choose between selling out my teammates and not selling books?

I refuse to do that. I was an adult when I made the choice to take Adderall. Nobody held a gun to my head. I took the first pill. And the ones after that. I can't blame anyone for any of my actions. I am now ready to talk about my personal experience, but I refuse to force any other guy's hands.

I was also told to be very careful about sharing my faith in this book. Apparently, that's just not politically correct and might offend someone. Supposedly, sharing my faith would kill book sales as well.

Needless to say, I called hogwash on all that. And I did not use a literary agent.

Ryan sat me down and gave me the skinny. He made it sound pretty easy. Apparently, all I had to do was ask the trainers for a form to submit to a doctor. A quick exam later, and I would be set with a prescription.

I didn't waste any time. I sought out a club trainer the first chance I got and filled out the form right then and there. I wanted to get this train rolling ASAP.

The adrenaline, joy, and excitement didn't end with the game. I was in such a state of bliss, I didn't want to (and couldn't) turn it off.

I was so glad it was a day game. Day games are great. Once you're done, you basically have the whole night ahead of you. So I rounded up some teammates and made plans for a nice dinner to commiserate our defeat.

I had always enjoyed a beer or two right after a game, and I usually downed a few before even hitting the shower. On this day, the thought of having a beer was absolute music to my ears. As I popped open the first can, it felt like I was drinking the most amazing beer in the world. It tasted so good. I had never realized just how refreshing and tasty a Bud Light could be.

Now that I had chugged a couple, for some reason I desperately felt the need to smoke a cigarette. Not just any cigarette, mind you, but a menthol. That was just weird to me. Up to this point in my life, I would only smoke the occasional cigarette to enhance my buzz and had never been a dipper. Never even gave tobacco much thought really. Now I was desperate for a Marlboro Menthol!

One of the clubhouse attendants hooked me up. I retreated to the laundry room to take a drag with an ice-cold brew in my hand. The first drag of that cigarette was epic. Just like the beer, I had never known a cigarette could taste *that* good. Every major sense in my body—taste, touch, sound, sight, smell—was at an extreme level of euphoria. *How could this drug be bad?* I thought to myself. At that moment, I sincerely felt that if everyone on the planet were on Adderall, the world would be a much better place.

I can't remember the name of the restaurant where we ate. Any Chicagoan will tell you that you can just throw a dart at a map of the city and hit an incredible place to eat. I would have to agree; I've never had a bad meal there. But as I sat staring at the menu, I realized I wasn't hungry at all.

I hadn't eaten since 11 a.m., right before I had downed the Adderall. I should have been famished by now, almost eight hours and nine full innings later. But I wasn't. Everything on the menu looked like tofu to me, except for the beer section. The beers were going down like Gatorade. I was putting a beer down every 10 minutes that entire dinner, and I didn't even feel drunk. In fact, the more I drank, the more heightened my sense of being became. I have since learned that Adderall makes it hard to realize just how much you have had to drink. Apparently, I was playing Russian roulette with alcohol poisoning every night I combined Adderall with alcohol.

I *knew* I had to eat something, so I forced down some kind of chicken dish. I had such cottonmouth that it was hard to make saliva to get the food down. The beer tasted fantastic, but I just had no desire to eat, and every bite felt like a kid must feel when his mom makes him eat all the broccoli on his plate.

Those who know me will tell you that I love to eat. Eating was normally one of my favorite things to do in this world besides sex and sleeping. This newfound distaste for food was new to me.

We had a great time at dinner, and the new Adderall-infused Aubrey was the life of the party. Dinner ended, and most of the guys were ready to head back to the hotel to get some rest. Normally, I would have been right there alongside them, but that night I wanted to keep going. I just couldn't turn off my brain. I wanted more stimuli. I was craving more alcohol, music, and atmosphere.

I managed to coerce one teammate to join me, and we found a nice little nightclub just a few blocks away. Chicago is definitely not lacking in amazing nightlife, and this place was no different. It was hopping. I must have downed at least another six beers, and we closed that place down before heading back to the hotel, a short cab ride away.

It was weird. I was definitely buzzed, not wasted, and still fully alert.

I swung through the revolving doors into the Westin lobby, the hum of the street sweepers along Michigan Avenue behind me. I paused for a second. The hotel bar was dead. It was now pushing 2:30 a.m. I should have been exhausted. But it felt like I had just woke up!

I lay on the bed staring at the ceiling. Mind racing. Normally, I would be laying there missing my wife and kid, feeling sorry for myself. Not tonight. Tonight, I saw myself playing well into my 40s. I was so excited I just couldn't turn my mind off. I replayed the day's game in my head, play by play, wondering how the hell I went 0-for-4. Counting sheep had never worked for me. And replaying the game wasn't working tonight either.

I found myself thinking, *How could just one little pill make such a difference in my attitude? How could I suddenly feel excited to be playing baseball again?* I was convinced that Adderall was going to be the savior I needed. The only way I could save my career.

I tossed and turned. I knew I had had at least 15 beers that night, and normally with that much booze running through my system I would pass out as soon as my head hit the pillow. But my brain was still trying to steal second base. After what seemed like an eternity, I could see the sun peeking through the shades in my room. The promise of another morning.

I finally drifted off to sleep.

I awoke that morning and almost had a heart attack. The alarm clock said it was 10 a.m.! I still had to pack my bag and get it to the hotel lobby for the travel secretary by 11 a.m. Plus, I had to shower, put my suit on, and make the team bus that I knew wouldn't wait for me. I had to get to the field! Most of the guys had already cabbed over to the stadium hours ago. Most likely, it would be just me and the team secretary on the bus. I remember feeling a sense of urgency, but the crazy thing was I wasn't in a panic, just in a heightened state of misery. I felt so melancholy, depressed even!

Shockingly, I wasn't hungover, even though I had consumed enough alcohol to tranquilize a horse. What I felt was different. A sort of hopelessness. I had never felt this low. The best way I can think to describe it is through a movie I saw a few years ago.

In the movie, *Limitless*, Eddie Mora (played by Bradley Cooper) takes a pill that's supposed to let him access all of his brain. On this drug, he becomes a superhuman version of himself. The only problem is that the next morning when he wakes up, he feels more miserable than ever. The only way for him to get back to feeling normal again is to pop another pill.

Well, that's what I felt like headed to the field that day. I knew I could never reproduce that Adderall high naturally. I felt like the only chance I had to feel somewhat like myself was to take another pill, and I had to do that ASAP. I could feel every bump and pothole the bus hit. The normal city noise and traffic sounded and felt like a jackhammer chipping away at my skull.

The minute I stepped into the clubhouse, I hit Ryan up for another Adderall. He kindly obliged, and I wasted no time washing it down. I wasn't even out of my street clothes, and I was already primed and ready, anxious for the high to hit. The high I had instantly fallen in love with the day before. The vicious cycle had begun.

I had a problem. On one hand, I absolutely loved playing baseball again on Adderall. But on the other, I had already witnessed firsthand what kind of guy this would turn me into off the field. I was torn. One side of the coin spelled absolute misery, living life and playing ball with no joy or excitement. My mind was made up. I had to have Adderall if I was going to save my career.

The paperwork and red tape seemed to drag on forever. It sure wasn't as easy as Ryan had made it sound. Finally, after what seemed like weeks, came the day where I would get in front of a doctor in downtown Baltimore.

I wasn't sure what to expect walking into his office that day. I sat in a small room, waiting for what seemed like an hour. The doctor walked in, and at first I didn't realize this was the specialist who would be prescribing this stuff to me. He was obese, talked with a slow drawl, and had a disheveled look about him. I knew immediately he wasn't on the stuff! I've had the "pleasure" of seeing a few psychiatrists in my life. This one got me on Adderall. The others I'd meet a few years later.

I fidgeted a little, but I should have known better. The whole experience felt like I was stealing candy from a baby. No one checked my pulse, blood pressure, or shoved a wooden stick down my throat. All the questions he asked me were layups. Basically, it wasn't a matter of whether I would get Adderall, more a matter of how many milligrams I wanted. He cut straight to the chase. He obviously knew why I was there and asked, "So Aubrey, a lot people that come to see me start out with 20 milligrams. But you're a big guy. You want to try 40?" I paused for a minute to contemplate. I had a feeling that this was pretty easy to score around the league, and wondered how many other guys were secretly walking around feeling as invincible as I did. "I'll just start with 20 and go from there," I replied.

I was out of there in 10 minutes! Walking out of the office I remember thinking, *So many guys in the league are on this, maybe finally I can level the playing field!*

Just a few weeks for the league to approve my application, I thought. In the meantime, I still had my one strike sitting in my pocket, just in case. So I rolled the dice those weeks, and never got tested.

Again, I knew it would be a few weeks. But just like little Ralphie in *A Christmas Story*, checking the mailbox twice a day for days on end, anxiously waiting for Little Orphan Annie's secret decoder, I walked into the clubhouse every day, fully expecting to see a little clear orange bottle waiting for me, a bow on top.

Finally, the day came. It felt like Christmas.

CHAPTER THREE
DETROIT. ROCK CITY.

*"Good talent with a bad attitude
equals bad talent"*

–BILL WALSH

Summer, 90 degrees. Clear sky.

Monday afternoon. August 17th, 2009. I remember it well.

About a month had passed since I'd swallowed my first Adderall. I rolled out of bed around noon, pulling the curtains open, hoping for rain so I wouldn't have to play that day. Not a cloud in the sky. It was like any other summer day in Baltimore, Maryland. Hot as hell, humid, with no breeze.

The game the previous night was a disaster. The Anaheim Angels had pummeled us 17-8. I was aching mentally and physically from the dog days of summer. The two bottles of Cabernet I polished off by myself after that game didn't help any. My eyelids were heavy, and the booze was having its way with my head and stomach.

Damn, I was tired of losing!

Maybe a long cold shower will wake me up, I thought. It didn't. I slowly dragged down the stairs of our quaint, little four-story townhouse we had purchased three years earlier. Baubi had been up and running for the past six hours taking care of our little one-year-old Jayce. I could tell she was overwhelmed and in absolutely no mood to even look at me. I dug out a bowl and poured myself some cereal.

After finishing off my breakfast of champions, I kissed Baubi good-bye, and hugged Jayce on my way out the door. I hopped on my bike and rode the two miles through the bustling downtown of Baltimore to Camden Yards. I normally loved that ride, especially on nice days. That quick fifteen minutes was usually just the perfect length for me to unwind a little, take some scenery in, and get ready for the chaos awaiting me at the field. It was a little harder, however, when I felt like this. I reluctantly pedaled to the field, taking my sweet time.

I arrived at the field and headed toward my locker to pop my 'better mood' pill, I spotted manager Dave Trembley sitting in my locker chair. "Follow me, Huffy," he said. He got up and headed toward his office. His look didn't give anything away. He didn't look mad or happy. I couldn't get a read on what this could be about. *Uh-oh*, I wondered. What did I do *this* time?

He swung his office door open. My gaze immediately met with Andy MacPhail's, general manager of the Orioles. He sat there on the couch with a confident grin on his face, as if he'd just made a savvy front-office move. My intuition immediately told me: *I've been traded!* The question was: Where?

Andy gave me his best "thanks for everything you've done" speech, then delivered the answer I had been waiting for. "Aubrey," he said happily, "we made the move to trade you to Detroit."

Getting traded brings a mixed bag of emotions. Part of you feels rejected, like a failure. Not appreciated. But the other part of you feels honored to be desired by someone else. I took it as a compliment, especially when I found out I would be going to the Tigers, a contending team. I was so excited to get out of Baltimore. Don't get me wrong, I enjoyed my teammates and loved the beautiful ballpark. I was just so sick of losing, and the Orioles were not even close to a playoff-caliber team.

I had to be in Detroit the next day to report for duty.

My mind went off on a roller-coaster ride. Thoughts of all that had to be done to move our little family hundreds of miles quickly began to flood my thoughts. *This would definitely put a lot of pressure on Baubi.* She was already overwhelmed with the long season and basically being a single parent. Now she would have to also handle much of the move.

I sprang into action and got busy packing my locker. I spent 20 minutes dishing out hugs and well-wishes to all my now-former teammates. My brothers for the past two and half years. I would be sad for a minute, then the gravity of my reality would hit: *I'm going to be in a playoff race!*

I glanced back at the clubhouse one final time on my way out the door, soaking up all I could for my memory bank. I knew I'd never see it again.

Now I had to tell Baubi. *No way I can tell her over the phone!*

I couldn't fit all my junk in my backpack for the bike ride back home. When you're making $10 million a year, a $1,000 bike is irrelevant, so I gave it to one of the rookies, and called a cab home. *One less thing to haul to Detroit*, I thought.

Because of the trade, I didn't even suit up or think about the game that day. I was still in my street clothes as I got out of the cab with my stuff in a box. How was I going to break this to my wife? The irony was that just the night before she was telling me how much she loved the view from our townhouse, the great location right on the harbor next to Federal Hill. And how much she enjoyed taking Jayce on the water ferry to Fells Point and Little Italy. "I really enjoy living in this area," she had said.

My wife has always been a trouper when it comes to the grind of moving from city to city, so I was confident she would be able to handle the news I was about to hit her with. She was sitting on the couch folding laundry and could obviously tell something big had just happened. Being a major league ballplayer's wife requires you to be able to move anywhere at the drop of a hat. I didn't even have to say anything as I walked toward her. She knew right away and asked with nervous anticipation, "Where we headed?"

Her face fell flat when I told her it was Detroit. She felt the same way as I did about that city. Although rich with baseball tradition, a gorgeous stadium, and a rabid fan base, it was not the ideal place to live or raise a kid. The downtown area was basically a ghost town, with the majority of the buildings boarded-up, looking like they should have been condemned long ago. Even on a gorgeous sunshine-laden day midweek, there were very few people walking around except for a bunch of unsavory characters looking for their next high. The only places that seemed to be happening were the downtown casinos. I knew we'd have to look well outside the city for a new place to call home. No more riding a bike to the stadium for me!

The next 24 hours were a blur. Again, my emotions ranged from nervous excitement, to joy, to feeling somehow betrayed. For a few moments each hour I would have to constantly remind myself, *This is what I signed up for. Plus, I'm making great money.* Being released or traded goes with the territory. Change is good. I have always embraced change. It can be uncomfortable, but I had always believed that in order to grow as a human being, you have to learn to get comfortable being uncomfortable.

It's always exciting arriving for your first day on a new team, not knowing what to expect. The cab driver taking me from the airport to Comerica Park happened to have the local sports talk radio station on. The subject? The arrival of Aubrey Huff. Caller after caller expressed their excitement for my arrival to solidify the middle of the Tigers batting order. I felt an immediate pride and a very strong sense of responsibility. I was now part of a contending team and had to earn my stripes immediately. The pressure to perform was mounting.

Even as a seasoned veteran, I felt a rush of nervous excitement walking into the clubhouse. I walked in with my head high, chest out, oozing with confidence. Inside, however, I felt really nervous taking in a new environment.

My locker was right next to the longest-tenured Tiger veteran, Brandon Inge. Brandon and I had met over the course of our careers and knew of each other because we shared agents. He was an old-school ballplayer who played the game with everything he had. I had a lot in common with him, and he made me feel right at home. He walked me around and introduced me to all the guys. It felt good to be introduced to a team the right way; meeting every player and clubhouse staff attendant on the first day. I felt like I would fit right into this organization.

After all the pleasantries with the Tigers players, I was called into the manager's office. Jim Leyland was in his 23rd big league season as a manager. The guy knew what he was doing. A three-time MLB Manager of the Year Award-winner. His crowning achievement: winning the 1997 World Series title managing the Florida Marlins. You could say I walked into his office feeling a little intimidated.

Jim was sitting at his desk in full uniform sucking down a Marlboro Red, and the minute I stepped into his office, I was almost knocked over by the smell of cigarette smoke.

"Hey Aubrey, have a seat. Welcome to the Tigers!" His voice had a deep monotone scratchy quality about it, no doubt the voice of a lifetime smoker. I sat down uncomfortably in my chair as he quickly launched into his expectations for me for the remainder of the season. "Aubrey we are excited to have you here," he said matter-of-factly. "We've been looking for a middle-of-the-order, left-handed bat all season. I also understand this is your first taste of a playoff drive?" His face was hard to read. He had that squinty Clint Eastwood–look about him. It seemed like he had done this a thousand times, and his expression was frozen somewhere between boredom and indifference.

"Yes, sir, it is. I couldn't be more thrilled to be here, Skip! How do you see me fitting into the lineup?" I asked.

He flipped the ash of his cigarette into a stainless steel ashtray that looked like it had been around longer than he had. He leaned back in his chair. "I see you hitting fifth behind Miguel Cabrera every day," he said. Definitely some first base, and DH. Maybe some third base and outfield, as well. In any case, you're my guy every day. So go out there, have fun, and enjoy your first playoff drive, son!"

The Detroit Tigers were in a comfortable first-place position in the American League Central when I showed up, and all the baseball experts had us as shoo-ins to win the division.

I walked out of his office obviously excited to be playing every day and hitting in the middle of a lineup that was expected to go deep into the playoffs.

My very first game as a Tiger I did, in fact, hit fifth, DH'ing behind the very dangerous Miguel Cabrera. The Seattle Mariners would be starting one of the best right-handed pitchers in baseball, Felix Hernandez. I was unusually nervous even with the 20-plus milligrams of Adderall doing their dance in my brain. All the pressure to make a good first impression and the fact that I was finally on a winner was almost too much for me to take. I wasn't used to this kind of pressure. Stands were packed full of Tigers fans cheering on our every move. I hadn't experienced this type of atmosphere up to this point in my big league career.

We won that game 5-3, and I finished a very modest 1 for 4. A sharp single up the middle off Felix Hernandez. With my work over, I breathed a huge sigh of relief, changed into street clothes, and cooled my throat with an ice-cold beer. Two beers later, my nerves had calmed down. The restlessness of the trade was starting to dissipate; and right at that moment, I felt right at home as a Detroit Tiger. For now!

Two games later, we faced Mariner left-handed pitcher Ryan Rowland-Smith. To my surprise, when I walked into the clubhouse to check the lineup, I was on the bench. I didn't read too much into it as I figured I must have struggled against him in the past. Or perhaps Jim wanted me to catch my breath after the whirlwind of the prior three days.

The very next game, we were up against the A's in Oakland. Once again, I warmed the bench. The A's threw left-handed pitcher Gio Gonzalez in the mix. Now I was beginning to get irritated. My new teammates were asking me what I did to piss off Jim Leyland. I was beyond confused. Wasn't it Jim himself just days earlier telling me I was going to play every day? That I was his guy, every day?

I had been an everyday player my entire life. And it looked as if I was already entrenched in the dreaded platoon-player role. Being a platoon-player meant I would only face right-handed pitchers, while sitting against left-handers, even though historically I had done quite well off southpaw pitchers.

My confusion grew, as did my bitterness. I coped the only way I knew how, by upping my dose of Adderall. *Gotta take the edge off.*

Deeper into that road trip in Anaheim, California, I was benched yet again against lefty Joe Saunders. *That's it. I have to have a conversation with Jim*, I thought. I immediately turned from the lineup card and headed toward Jim's office in full steam, clearly upset.

I knocked on the ajar glass-paneled door and walked in. I sucked in a lungful of cigarette smoke, "Can we chat, Skip?" The look he gave me gave every indication this was going to be an awkward conversation. "Jim, what the hell is going on?" My voice quivered as I struggled to maintain my cool. "I thought you said I was going to play every day," I continued.

"Um, no Aubrey, I never remember saying that," he stated aggressively. I was floored. *He is either lying or losing his memory in his old age*, I reasoned.

I continued, "Skip, I have been an everyday player my whole life, and have hit lefties very well in the past. I'm not really sure what my role is here. I thought I was brought in to be a difference-maker, not a platoon-player."

He replied, "Well Aubrey, I have to make sure I get everyone their at bats, and sometimes I have to sit you to make sure other guys stay sharp."

I knew then and there that this conversation was going nowhere. I sarcastically thanked him for his time, and walked out of his office even madder and more confused than when I had walked in. *Why the hell was I traded here in the first place?*

You can guess how the rest of that season went for me. The Tigers had spent 146 days in first place that season. But the magic wouldn't last. We became the first team in Major League Baseball history to lose a three-game lead with four games left to play. We won the final game of the regular season, however, and found ourselves in a tie with the Minnesota Twins who came out of nowhere that September playing red-hot baseball. It would come down to a one-game, winner-take-all matchup: game 163, to be played in Minnesota. The winner would go to the playoffs. The loser would go home.

We landed in Minnesota the night before the big game, boarded the team bus and headed to the hotel, a nervous excitement in the air. I found out on the bus that the Twins would be throwing a right-handed pitcher, Scott Baker.

I don't think I slept that whole night. I was so excited for the game. *Maybe this was the moment I was traded over for. It was destiny!* After all, I only played against right-handers, so I would be one of the guys playing in a do-or-die, playoff-type game!

I was already picturing myself hitting a game-winning home run to send the Tigers to the playoffs. I would be forever remembered in Tigers lore. I had waited my whole life for this moment. The opportunity to play in a big game and the chance to go to the playoffs for the first time in my career. I couldn't wait to pop the champagne! But I was getting way ahead of myself.

I was one of the first players to race excitedly to the lineup card the next morning. It was October 7th, 2009. A Wednesday. I looked right at the middle of the lineup card where my name would be, fully expecting to see it. Nope. I looked lower, and lower. Nothing. I finally glanced at the bench players and there I was: Huff. Now I have been kicked in the balls a couple times in my life quite literally, and this felt way worse. I was sick to my stomach with anger. I stormed to my locker, popped open my pill jar, and shoved down two pills of Adderall. That's 40 milligrams if you're counting. I had never done that much in one sitting. But I didn't care. I was embarrassed, confused, and in a state of rage that is hard to explain. I sat there at my locker not engaging anyone. I stared down at the floor like an eight year-old whose mom didn't let him get his favorite toy from Toys "R" Us. I didn't move. I sat there frozen until it was time for batting practice.

It took everything I had to get suited up and go take batting practice with my team. Nobody on the team said a word to me that day. The expression on my face said it all. I was walking around red-faced, nostrils flared, mouth closed tight, and eyebrows pointed down as much as physically possible. Not necessarily the attitude you would want to see from a player before a game of this magnitude.

The Adderall was in full effect just in time for the first pitch. My rage lurked just beneath the surface, ready to blow at any minute. But even with it pushing against the rev limiter like it was, it was easily surpassed by the excitement in the stadium. The atmosphere was electric in the Metrodome that day with 54,088 excited fans. Absolutely deafening! I had never in all of my life heard such an ear-splitting noise. And that made me even more enraged. I was infuriated that I was missing out on such a big game! I sat at the end of the bench the entire game, arms crossed. Occasionally, I would clap when we made a good play, just so I would seem like a good teammate.

I know this may sound sick, but it's the truth. As soon as I saw my name on the bench that day, I found myself secretly hoping we would lose, just so Jim Leyland wouldn't get the credit. I hoped this, knowing the disappointment it would cause the guys on the team whom I genuinely liked. Looking back at it now, I realize how childish it sounds. I also now realize that Jim was no doubt doing what he felt was right for the team. I couldn't have made his job any easier being the baby I was.

I wanted to blame him for my poor performance at the time. I wasn't man enough to accept the fact that I was just not producing when I did get my at bats. Like a bona fide loser, I made excuses. Jim had been around the block a few times; he had probably seen hundreds of guys like me. I hate to say this, but as much as I wanted to play, Jim made the right call. The bench was where I belonged. Adderall threw any rationale I had out the window. Looking back, I couldn't feel more embarrassed for my attitude.

This game was living up to its billing. Everyone in the stadium was on the edge of their seat as we headed into the 10th inning tied-up at 5. I was sitting at the end of the bench with my helmet next to me, batting gloves on, bat in my hands just in case I got a chance to pinch hit. Sure enough, Jim called from the end of the bench, "Aubrey, you're hitting for Ramirez." A rush of adrenaline shot through my body. *This is it! My chance at being the hero. This was why I was brought here.* All the negativity could be erased in this moment. Let's win this thing!

With one out and nobody on, I dug into the left handed batter's box with one mission, hit a homerun. The pitcher for the Twins was Jesse Crain. To my disappointment I was hit in the leg by an 0-2 fastball, limping my way to first. To top it all off Don Kelly pinch ran for me. Back to the bench for me. A miserable end to my stellar night. Ironically enough this pretty much summed up my time with Detroit.

Bottom of the 12th, a 5-5 game. The game was now pushing against the five-hour mark. The tension in the stadium was at a tipping point. Any pitch could be the last.

The Twins had one out. Runners at first and second. Alexi Casilla stepped up to the plate. And just like that, after five grueling hours, Alexi put an end to the heart-palpitating game for everyone with a walk-off single to right field, driving in the runner from second.

The roar of the crowd in the Metrodome was deafening. My heart broke for my teammates, knowing how hard they had worked that season, how hard they had fought the last 12 innings. But deep inside my gut, I wanted to scream out jubilantly with the crowd. The Twins had just put an end to my misery in Detroit.

CHAPTER FOUR
A .357 MAGNUM

"The tragedy of life is not death,
but what we let die inside of us
while we live."

—NORMAN COUSINS

My pain in Detroit for a little over a month pales in comparison to the lifetime of anguish caused by my father's murder. Reality is, we will all have to deal with the death of a loved one sooner or later. For me, it came sooner in life. December 15th, 1983, at 4:15 p.m., to be exact. I was six years old.

My mother had rushed home early from work that day, worried and curious as to why my grandfather wanted her home immediately. She hurried through the front door, hair still messy from a hard day's work, throwing a pained glance at my sister, Angie, and me as we sat in the living room in front of the TV.

My grandparents moved in close and spoke softly to her where she stood, just inside the front door. She leaned back against the frame of the door, eyes locked in on my grandfather's. Whatever he whispered made her face turn a beet red, and caused tears to stream down her face in an uncontrollable flood. I sat frozen on the couch, not sure what to do or say.

Just 30 minutes earlier, the phone had rung. A call that would interrupt my favorite cartoon and instantly change my life.

It was Christmas break. Here I was, just five days before my seventh birthday, with no responsibilities or worries. My whole world was in the now. I didn't care about the past, nor did I fret about my future. I was simply at peace in the present with no schedule to follow, and no fear. A feeling of absolute happiness and wonder I have spent my entire adult life trying desperately to recapture. Life was easy, and the future was full of magical possibilities.

My four-year-old sister, Angela, was quietly playing with her dolls in the corner. My grandfather, Rufus Horn, was reading the paper as he did daily for hours. My grandmother, Meda, stood at the kitchen sink, apron tied around her waist, washing dishes from lunch. She always seemed to be washing dishes.

The old yellow rotary phone on the wall rudely pierced through the quiet of the early afternoon with an obnoxious ring. As I was watching *The Transformers*, I remember being annoyed that it was interfering with my ability to hear what Optimus Prime was saying. My grandfather strolled over and answered in his very deep Southern accent, "Hello." The five-foot-long curly cord hung loosely from the receiver, dangling at his waist. He listened for a moment. His shoulders sank and his demeanor changed almost instantly. He seemed to be very stoic in his responses, "Uh-huh, uh-huh, I see. I'll notify the family. Thank you."

He hung up, a look of confusion on his face, and walked over to my grandmother. She was drying the dishes by now. I heard hushed voices, followed moments later by the sound of shattering glass on the kitchen floor, and a sorrow-filled scream, "Oh, Lord, NO!"

I rushed over, desperate to find out what had just happened. My poor grandma sat at the kitchen table, white as a ghost. My grandfather stood by her side, hand on her shoulder.

"What happened?" I asked. I was convinced my grandma had cut herself on some sharp glass. My grandpa's response was calm, "Let's call your mother first and have her come home so we can have a conversation as a family." With this, he got back on the phone, called my mother at Winn-Dixie, and implored her to come home right away. "No, the kids are okay," and not to worry about them, he told her.

I looked, but couldn't see any blood anywhere. I desperately tried to console my grandma who was crying uncontrollably for... I had no idea what!

After what seemed like a lifetime, I heard my mom's car pull up and her car door slam shut. She appeared at the door a few moments later, my grandparents breaking the news, whatever it was, in hushed tones.

My mom's face was ashen. Eyes swollen. Mini-rivers washing mascara down each side of her pretty face. She shuffled slowly into the living room and sank into a cushion next to me on the couch. My grandpa picked up my sister and joined us.

I remember the scent of that moment. It smelled like a combination of Old Spice and flowery-scented sweat. I felt my mom's warm embrace. Her tears dampened my hair as she fought back the lump in her throat. She held back her tears just long enough to explain in a sad, monotone voice that my father would not be coming home ever again. He was in a better place. He had just died, and was now in heaven.

That was it.

I went right back to watching *The Transformers* on television. A blank, unemotional stare on my face. I remember thinking, *He was never here anyway.* Even as a six year-old boy, I knew it was very strange that I did not shed a single tear that night.

Aubrey Lewis Huff Jr. was a Texan through and through. He loved to fish, hunt, and play the guitar. So I was told. I don't remember much about him. Not even the sound of his voice. My sister and I had never really been told what he was like, or what kind of father or husband he was. Just that—he liked to hunt, fish, and play guitar. A shroud of mystery surrounded the topic of my father around our household. We just did not talk about him, and whenever I probed my mom for details, she would seem very uncomfortable and change the subject right away. I figured it must have been very hard for her to talk about since he had died so tragically, so I never dug deeper. It was not until years later that my mom would fill in a few details for me, explaining the circumstances surrounding his death and about their relationship around that time.

For reasons I would not discover until much later in life, my father was living in Abilene, Texas, when he died, a two-hour drive from our home in Mineral Wells. He had been living and working as the staff electrician at The Royal Orleans apartment complex there. My father's sister, Mary Rodriguez, said that just before his death, my dad was acting suspiciously, constantly staring out between the window blinds as if to check if anyone had followed him home. Apparently he had become very paranoid. As it turns out, he had good reason to be.

According to the *Abilene Reporter-News* December 16th, 1983:

A man and woman were shot to death at The Royal Orleans Apartments Thursday, and moments later police arrested the woman's estranged husband. Kerri Jo Hughes, 23, and Aubrey Lewis Huff Jr., 30, died at the scene.

Police arrested Travis Ray Hughes, of Comanche, moments after the shooting. Two witnesses identified Hughes by name as the man who fired the shots, police said.

Officer Bryan Smith arrived on the scene to find, "a white male lying face down in the doorway on the east side of the office and a white female lying behind a desk almost directly in front of the door."

There was nothing peaceful about the way my father left this Earth.

He was headed to the front office to clock out for the day when he heard a couple arguing very loudly. As he approached the couple to defuse the situation, Travis Hughes pulled a gun on him. A .357 Magnum. My dad's first reaction was to slap the gun away, and as he did, it went off, striking him in the hip, and dropping him to the floor. Hughes then turned to his estranged wife who was cowering behind the desk, shooting her once in the chest, and once in the head. He killed her instantly. My dad lay on the floor bleeding profusely from the initial hit.

According to court documents, Hughes then pointed the gun toward complex manager Janee Jackson. My dad leaped up and shoved her out of the way, tackling Hughes, and knocking the gun out of his hand again. The two wrestled around on the floor for a few minutes, but my father's wound made the match an unfair one. Hughes won the battle, grabbed the gun, and cowardly shot my dad in the back of the head, killing him instantly as he stumbled toward the door. He lay in a pool of blood, right where he fell. He was just 30 years old.

Travis Ray Hughes was sentenced to 99 years in a Texas prison for the murder of his ex-wife, and 10 years for the involuntary manslaughter of my father. He is still serving that sentence.

Questions were asked at the trial as to the relationship between my father and Travis Hughes' estranged wife, Kerri. During the trial, Travis testified that he felt my father and Kerri were having an affair. I often wonder, *Were they? Why else would he be checking outside his window, acting paranoid?* I will never truly know. And for a long time, that hurt deeply.

Despite that, I was and still am incredibly proud of my dad, knowing that he saved a life. He was a hero in my book, and that has been the way I have chosen to remember him to this day. He died committing a very selfless act. My father may not have been the most attentive husband or father, but one thing I'm sure of was that he did love us. I just don't think he knew how to show it.

My aunt Mary told me that in the weeks leading up to his death, my father began to feel deep regret for the things he had done in his life and the people he had hurt. He told her he had started going to church, and after one of the services he was moved so much that he gave his life to Christ.

A note he wrote to my mom just a week before he died confirms his change of heart in his final weeks on this Earth. It was a letter filled with sincerity and love. In it he asks for forgiveness for all he had done to her, my sis, and me. I cry tears of joy when I think that maybe, just maybe, my dad is waiting for me to join him in heaven one day.

I believe we have an epidemic on our hands here in the Western world, and especially America. It breaks my heart to hear about kids all across our amazing country losing their way, having sex in junior high, turning to drugs and alcohol to ease their burdens. I hate hearing about so many kids who are so stressed about school that they are suicidal. Bullying is at an all-time high. Kids are stealing, breaking and entering, joining violent gangs, and even killing. I am sure none of this is news to you.

According to Wikipedia, 63 percent of kids who commit suicide are raised in fatherless homes, as are 90 percent of all homeless and runaway children. So, too, are 85 percent of children who exhibit behavior disorders, and a full 80 percent of rapists with anger problems. The statistics are staggering. 71 percent of all high school dropouts and 85 percent of all youth in prison today do not grow up with a father in their lives.

I know what it's like to grow up without a father, so this is a topic that I am passionate about. The scariest statistic of all for me is that according to the U.S. Department of Census, 43 percent of children in the USA are living in a home without a father right now. 43 percent! That's almost half the kids in America! My prayer is that the men of our generation will step up and take an active role in the lives of our children.

I glanced away from the TV for a minute, and watched as my mom got up from the couch, eyes still swollen, shoulders hunched over. She gave me a genuine, loving smile, as if to say, "Everything is going to be okay." That was all that was said about my father for a long time.

I was fatherless at the age of six, the prime age for a dad to start pouring love, knowledge, strength, courage, and wisdom into me. My mom's parents stepped up big time to fill the void left by my father's death. They practically raised my sister and me, and had a huge influence on who I would become as a man. My grandparents even profoundly impacted my baseball career.

Rufus and Meda Horn never seemed comfortable sharing their faith, but the way they loved on Angie and me, and the way they acted around us and others, had a deeper impact on me than any preacher I had come across.

I loved my grandfather's humble, quiet, soft-spoken demeanor and very dry, witty sense of humor. Growing up in Scranton, Texas, a tiny town 40 miles east of Abilene, my grandpa learned how to farm at a young age. Just like many Texan men his age, he knew how to live off the land without relying on handouts or help from the outside world. That hardscrabble attitude helped him become a leader on his basketball team at Scranton High. His six-foot, two-inch, 210-pound stature didn't hurt either.

He met my grandmother at a high school dance, but they didn't marry until five years later. Meda was every bit of five-three, maybe 110 pounds; she was very direct and knew how to get what she wanted. She was raised a seamstress, and was also a standout on her high school basketball team.

It would be 16 years before they had children. Doctors told them they may never conceive. But just after they stopped trying to have kids, my uncle Audie, and two years later my mother, Fonda, were born. I can never forget my mom's birthday: September 11th, 1955.

Like her father, my mom loved basketball too. I'm amazed I didn't pursue that sport instead of baseball. But the seed for my baseball passion was planted in the months following my dad's death, and it took deep roots. My grandmother, in particular, was a rabid Texas Rangers baseball fan. She would have every game on the television or radio, and she always let me stay up late until the last out was recorded. Even today when I need to go back to a loving, comforting moment in my life, I often go back in my mind to my grandparents' house all those years ago. I still remember sitting in her frail lap, being held tight in her arthritic hands that smelled like Bengay. I can't remember a time in my young life when I felt more loved.

Watching and listening to the Rangers inspired me. I desperately needed someone to play catch with. Someone to throw to me so I could learn to swing the bat. Most kids I knew had their fathers to help them. That wasn't an option for me. So my 69 year-old grandma stepped up to the plate, a three-pack of wiffle balls, and a fat orange bat in hand. A $3.99 Target special.

Our stadium was the beautifully manicured, seventy-feet-long and forty-feet-wide side yard of their modest 1,100-square-foot, three-bedroom home in Mineral Wells, Texas. My grandma would wind up the pitch underhand, and I would swing with everything I had. The plastic-on-plastic smack of the bat hitting the ball would be music to my ears as I watched the balls sail over the chain link fence to my left, out onto the street. My poor grandmother would limp out into the street to retrieve the balls over and over again, fighting neighborhood traffic.

We practiced like this several times until one day she had a brilliant idea. Why chase the balls when she could have them come back to her? So she turned me around and made me bat left-handed. This way, she thought, the balls would simply hit the house to my right and ricochet back to her. No more dodging traffic.

I write right-handed, throw right-handed, I even play golf right-handed. But I bat left-handed. Now you know why.

I don't know if I could have gone as far playing baseball hitting right-handed. And there is just no way my grandmother could have known what a huge impact that simple switch would have on my career decades later.

My grandpa didn't speak all that often. When he did, I sat up and listened. I looked up to him, and he was always there with advice whenever I needed it or asked for it. He wasn't the type of guy to sit me down and talk to me about the birds and the bees as I got older, as a matter of fact, I never got *that* talk. He wasn't the most affectionate man either. I don't remember getting a hug from him too often. But his firm Texas handshake each time he greeted me, followed by an intense respectful stare into my eyes told me beyond a shadow of a doubt that he loved me. Rufus Horn was the one man in my life I could count on. He always made sure I got to where I needed to be on time. I never missed school, baseball practices, or after-school activities. And I was never waiting around for him to pick me up.

My grandparents were tough and accepted their lot in life. Even when my grandmother began getting dialysis for her kidneys, I didn't hear her complain about her situation or failing health. The last few months of her life were difficult, but again, she remained in great spirits and was so happy to see us visiting her in the hospital.

I showed up to the hospital for a visit one day before heading to the field for spring camp, and I couldn't believe the woman I saw lying there was my grandmother. The nurse had warned me that I should be prepared for what I was about to see, and that I should say my final good-bye. I was literally heartbroken walking through the door to her room. She lay there motionless, a pale purple, facial skin so sunken she looked like a skeleton, tubes and IVs all over her body. I knew right then she wouldn't make it past the night.

I sat in that flower-filled hospital room and held her cold, lifeless hand in mine. "Grandma, it's me, Aubrey." I felt her squeeze my hand ever so slightly. I knew the large tube down her throat wouldn't allow her to speak, so I asked her to squeeze my hand if she could hear. She did with all her might.

I tried to be strong. I swallowed hard and poured my heart out to her, telling her how much I loved her, and just how much she meant to me. I thanked her over and over for all the years of self-less dedication and love she had shown me and our family. I told her how much I looked up to her and appreciated her strength.

I attempted to comfort her by reminding her that she would soon be in paradise with Jesus, and even added a little humor, telling her to have my favorite dish of hers ready for me when I got there. Her famous fried then baked chicken. Her eyes closed, tears escaping, running down her face. A faint smile appeared as I sat there holding her hand.

I took one last turn on my way out of the room, tears in my eyes. I knew this would be the final time I saw my grandmother alive. Meda Horn passed away the next morning, February 3rd, 2004, at the age of 89.

My grandfather had lost his soulmate, and couldn't cope. He wandered around the house in his wheelchair asking when Meda was going to come home. I remember on one particular occasion he attempted to open the door of my car going seventy down the highway. He was absolutely losing it mentally.

I saw him roll his wheelchair out the door, no idea where he was, as I delivered an emotional eulogy for my grandmother. My sister had to go out and wheel him back in. The sadness of that situation still weighs on me today. We had no choice but to check him into a retirement home with round-the-clock care soon after that. He refused to eat and would not leave the house. I could tell he was ready to join his soulmate of 67 years.

I visited him in the hospital two months later. He looked really bad and the constant winces on his face told me he was in a lot of pain. I had barely set foot in his room when he yelled out to me, "Hey you, I want out of here!" He didn't recognize me, and even though I tried to explain to him who I was, it just wasn't registering. All he kept telling me was that he was in pain, and asked could I help him. I tried desperately to hold back tears, but just couldn't.

My grandfather was the only male presence in my life, and now I knew I was about to lose him, too. I fought through the tears long enough to say all I could say to him. How much I loved him and how much he meant to me. I couldn't look back as I closed the door and walked down the hallway crying. All I could hear was his pained voice. Words that haunt me to this day. "Help me! Help me!" My grandfather, Rufus Horn, passed away that night, April 14th, 2004, at the age of 91.

Losing her main sources of strength in her life within six weeks of each other was incredibly hard on my mother. The only thing that made the eulogy I delivered at my grandpa's funeral easier was knowing he and his bride of almost 70 years were together once again. No longer in pain.

My grandparents' legacy of selfless love may not have changed the world, but it certainly transformed mine. They had shown me how we all have just one chance to leave a lasting legacy in this life, and I didn't want to blow it. I *had to* succeed at the career they had helped me launch.

The pain of Detroit was behind me. The next chapter of my life could not come soon enough.

CHAPTER FIVE
HIT ME!

*"Addiction is the only prison
where the locks are on the inside."*

—ANONYMOUS

I went into that offseason a free agent convinced I was a bad luck charm, a cancer, if you will. I distinctly remember this overwhelming feeling I would *never* taste the playoffs.

The offseason is a time to recharge. To give your body a rest from the wear and tear, and the drugs. But I continued my Adderall use every day. Baubi was all over me to start contributing around the house, and finally become an involved, loving father to Jayce. But I simply couldn't. I was stuck in my own despair. Still disappointed in how my previous season had played out. Blaming everybody else.

I have never sat down and studied Adderall's side effects in those four-page magazine ads with lettering so small you need a magnifying glass to read it. As an expert witness and user for almost three years, however, I have my theories. The biggest thing Adderall did for me was enhance my natural personality traits. I believe that a sensitive person will be unable to resist the urge to cry on Adderall. And that if you have a very addictive personality, it will put you in rehab faster than you can read this next sentence. Angry people plus Adderall equals prison time.

I am not naturally sensitive, addicted to stuff, or angry. I am however, a very compulsive guy by nature. When I get bored, I'll instinctively do whatever is on my mind without any thought of how my actions may impact me or anyone else. I'll go buy something really expensive without doing any research. And I believe that Adderall transformed me into the most compulsive person that ever walked planet earth.

Case in point: One beautiful Saturday morning in Tampa, Florida. I am not sure what set me off, but I woke up feeling inspired. I decided I wanted to put up some Christmas lights for the holidays. So after my morning pill and coffee, off I went to Santa's Workshop in Clearwater, Florida. The plan was to get a few lights to put up, nothing crazy. The Adderall kicked into gear about the time I arrived at the store. It was nine a.m., and Mr. Hyde took over, ratcheting up my compulsiveness by a thousand percent. I spent three hours in that store, buying everything from giant, stuffed reindeers and polar bears for inside the house, to well over $4,000 worth of outdoor Christmas lights. When I was done decorating, the house looked better than Clark Griswold's house in *National Lampoon's Christmas Vacation*.

Christmas lights were just the beginning. I developed another compulsive habit courtesy of Adderall that offseason: blackjack. I was never really a gambler or had any interest in gambling of any kind until that time in my life. Oh sure, I'd play the occasional roulette wheel or maybe $10 hands to kill time on the rare occasion. But I never considered myself to have a gambling problem.

Now, I found myself frequenting the Hard Rock Casino in Tampa five times a week to kill the boredom of the day. Sometimes I would win, most times I would lose. It has to be the dopamine levels or something that the drug pumps through your brain. Gambling was such an adrenaline rush, I just couldn't get enough. I would be out until three a.m., sometimes six in the morning, just sitting at the table by myself having hours of conversation with the dealers of the night. It was strange to me that I didn't want to be around anyone I knew when I was in that state. I enjoyed the isolation, the solitude. Now, years later, I think that maybe that was because deep down I didn't want my friends or family seeing what a complete mess I had become. But more on that later.

You would think that after a season like the one I had just had, I would be ready to get my life back together, get off the Adderall, and get busy working out to save my baseball career. Nope. It was quite the opposite for me. I was almost numb to the game. I truly was at a point in my life where I didn't care if I played one more inning. Baseball had become public enemy number one. I was sick of the misery, pain, and heartache the game was causing me. Deep down I was glad I was a free agent, essentially unemployed. I was secretly hoping a team wouldn't sign me, just so I could quietly ride off into the sunset, forgotten about, forever.

It was just after the New Year. I was thumbing through a newspaper, watching my coffee go cold. Baubi walked into the living room holding one of those little pregnancy test sticks. Of course, I knew what that meant! No need to look at the little red lines. Probably another miracle. Well, considering how much she hated even looking at me, much less touching me those days, *definitely* a miracle. I was excited, but not as excited as I should have been about our second child. Something inside me screamed out, *Great! Just more responsibility!* My first son, Jayce, was not even a toddler, and already I had pushed him away, making sure I had absolutely no relationship with him. Baubi did everything with and for him. She fed and bathed him, woke up in the middle of the night with him, spent hundreds of hours nurturing him each week like the amazing mother she was. She was basically a single parent, with me only occasionally chipping in to help. When I felt like it. And now, we were about to add another child to the mix. I found myself thinking, *Are we still gonna be married by the time our second child is born?*

Spring training was fast approaching, and I was still without a team. As a matter of fact, I hadn't gotten a single call. Probably a good thing since there was absolutely no way I would have been ready anyway. I only worked out maybe 30-minutes daily that offseason, barely breaking a sweat. I didn't once pick up a baseball bat to hit. Hardly the prep routine of a champion.

To fuel my blackjack compulsion, I decided to learn the art of card counting. I found a professional card counter online and hired him. I will call him *Ralph*. He lived all the way out on the other side of the country in California, and I paid his full airfare to Tampa. He patiently worked with me for the weekend, and taught me the basic gist of card counting. Now it was time to test my skills with a flight to Vegas. When I told Baubi I was going to Sin City, she actually looked happy to hear the news. I'm guessing she really wanted me out of the house.

It was late January 2010, and here I was in Vegas, jobless. I had invited my best friend and best-man at my wedding, Russ Jacobson, and another friend of mine, Alex Santos, along for the action that weekend. They had both played baseball with me at the University of Miami. Russ was a fellow redneck with all my same core values. Anyone who knows us will tell you we even have identical personalities. We looked so much alike on the baseball field that oftentimes people would get us confused. We had a lot in common and became best friends so fast that our mothers started calling us both their sons. Russ became more than just a friend that year. He became my brother. To this day we tell each other everything, and I can't even imagine going through life without him to confide in.

Alex is not only one of my best friends to this day, he is also my financial adviser. So obviously he wasn't thrilled I was there to gamble all my savings away. Ralph convinced me that I needed to take out $100,000 to get started with. My goal was to double that. I did very well for a couple of days; as a matter of fact, I won about $25,000 as Russ, Alex, and Ralph watched. Two of them in nervous horror.

Ralph had had all the fun he could, and decided he needed to get back home to California. So Russ, Alex, and I decided to stay one more night. The plan was to just hang. Something we had not done in years. We chatted at the Bellagio bar most of the night, sporadically making small bets at the blackjack tables, just enjoying each other's company.

Everything seemed to be going well until around 11 p.m. All of a sudden, the Adderall compulsiveness that had turned me into Clark Griswold a few months earlier kicked in with full force. I became obsessed with this feeling that I wanted to take the house down. I was insistent on hitting the VIP casino area to play big money against the advice of my good friends. They told me in no uncertain terms that they wanted no part of it. They went upstairs for the night. They were going to fly home early the next morning, and thought it best to try to get some sleep.

I pulled up a chair in the VIP area willing to put ten grand on the line. The dealer behind the table looked like a nice enough guy. I started out very modestly, with a single bet of $1,000.

Blackjack! I doubled my bet. Blackjack again! *This is gonna be a good run*, I thought to myself.

I was on a hot streak! Marlboro Menthol had become my cigarette of choice now every time I was high. I lit one up and took a drag. *It's time to get really aggressive. Finally take the house down.* I upped my bet from $1,000 a hand to all seven spots at the table at $1,000 each—$7,000 a hand! By this time, I was too plastered to count cards. I was running on dumb luck.

After about twenty hands, I stopped for a quick breather. I reached for another menthol and glanced down at the enormous pile of chips in front of me. To my amazement, I had amassed over $240,000 in plastic! I was ecstatic. I hadn't realized I was doing *that* well. It had happened so fast. I looked behind me. At least 20 people were behind a velvet rope cheering me on. I had my own personal waitress serving me endless Bud Lights. I was on a roll; I couldn't be beaten. Two pit bosses watched my every move with hawk-like eyes.

It was around three a.m. now, and I was still doing very well, winning more hands than I was losing. I was pushing almost 300 grand. Not bad considering I had started with $10,000! The phones started blowing up in the pit boss area. Not 30 seconds later, a beautiful, tall, busty brunette snuck under the velvet red rope and brought me a Bud Light. She sat down beside me to chat. She was very aggressive, "Hey handsome, I can tell you like to party. Want to come join me at the club? You won't be disappointed."

I was under the influence big time, but even so, I knew immediately what was going on. The hotel had obviously called in one of their "coolers" to throw me off my game. It was The Bellagio doing its very best to slow me down, and I was having none of it. I looked her straight in the eyes, and with a stern tone told her, "Thanks for the beer, but I'm not falling for this hustle.

Beat it!" Then I turned and looked right at one of the pit bosses, and with a smile on my face said, "I'm not falling for that one, buddy!" He gave me a devious smile back. I immediately looked up to the eyes in the sky, and shot them all the middle finger! I was invincible! I looked back down at the dealer. He winked at me and smiled. He was on my side. After all, I had probably tipped him 20 grand since I sat down!

The girl left, and I started to lose. The cooler strategy had worked. She had at least rubbed some bad luck on me, I figured. Thank goodness Russ came down to check on me right about then.

He saw all the chips in front of me, and said to me in the sternest voice I've ever heard him use, "Aubrey, that's enough! Let's cash out before you lose it all!" I was now down to about 200 grand, and my stockpile was falling at the rate of about $10,000 a minute. I was in such a high, drunk, aggressive state, I told him, "Piss off, Russ!" in a harsh tone that surprised even me. As a matter of fact, Russ told me later that I was so belligerent and rude to him that night, that he was really questioning our friendship after that trip. He couldn't take me anymore. It was one thing when we drank together, but it was a whole other thing when I was drunk *and* high.

Alex joined us in the VIP room a few minutes later, and when he, too, saw the $180,000 in chips in front of me, he almost dropped dead of a heart attack. He motioned over to Russ, and with a quick, fluid motion, they grabbed me by both arms and yanked me out of my seat, onto my feet. The room was spinning around me. I was so tanked that I couldn't stand or walk without Russ's help. I almost fell to the floor, but steadied myself long enough to haphazardly gather my chips. I felt my buddies drag me out of there.

The pit boss, relieved to be finally rid of me, escorted us out to the safe area, and helped us stash the chips in the casino safe for the night. Russ would tell me later that Alex had to walk behind me, picking up the countless $10,000 chips I was dropping all over the floor as I stumbled to the safe. He also told me that he and Alex had to literally carry my 215-pound carcass through the casino to the elevator because I had passed out just as the safe door slammed shut. To make matters worse, on the ride up in the elevator, I began pissing my pants. They threw me into bed fully clothed, completely dead to the world just before sunup.

I woke up the next day to a text around three p.m. Here I was lying in my Bellagio bed smelling like piss and feeling like I got hit by a truck. The text was from Russ, "Bud, it was great seeing you. But I have to tell ya, you're turning into someone I don't like all that much. I hope you can get your life turned around. You have a problem. I love ya, man! Oh, by the way don't forget about the 180 grand in the safe." *Oh damn! I would have totally forgotten about that,* I thought. *Maybe Russ is right. Maybe I do have a problem.*

Baubi was not at all impressed by my version of the events of the weekend. As I recounted my story, I could sense she was cold and distant. Not even me proudly showing her the 180 grand I had won could turn her frown upside down. She was numb to me and I had a feeling there wasn't much more she could take. Here she was pregnant, and with a one-year-old boy in tow. The last thing she needed was her husband acting like he was a child, struggling through a drugged-out midlife crisis!

It was the first week of February, just two weeks before spring training. Finally, I got a call from my agent. "Aubrey, we have a deal on the table. One year, three million dollars, with the San Francisco Giants. I think we should take it."

Wow! San Francisco was the last place I thought would come calling. I loved my trips as a visiting player to that city over the years. However, AT&T Park wasn't necessarily one of the most hitter-friendly parks in the league. San Francisco is where hitters' careers went to die. Ironically enough, my career was dying anyway, so I felt I should fit right in. I wasn't too thrilled at the prospect of being a Giant, nor was I thrilled at the contract. Just $3 million. I had just came off three consecutive years of making $10 million a year. This would be a huge pay cut. But what other choice did I have?

Before I was to sign on the dotted line, Brian Sabean, Giants general manager, called me. He was already at the Giants' spring training complex in Scottsdale, Arizona, and wanted to meet.

I flew out of Tampa the next day and was immediately escorted into Brian's office. Now pause for a moment and humor me. See if you can see me through the eyes of Brian Sabean as I walked in that afternoon. Picture me walking through his door. 34 years old, with frosted tip blond highlights in my Mohawk hairdo. Black diamond stud earring in my left ear. Rock star jacket. Over-the-top rock star jewelry around my neck and on my fingers. I looked like the front man for a rock band, not a baseball player!

The first thing he said to me was, "Damn, Aubrey, you're sure not what I expected." I was shocked to hear him say that. I asked him what he meant. "Honestly, I have heard from multiple sources around the league that you were a bit chubby and out of shape, and that you like to party. But by seeing you walk in, I can at least see you're in decent shape."

Now keep in mind, I hadn't done a single thing baseball-related all that offseason. I had, however, been high 24/7. And for me, Adderall wiped out my appetite. I was never hungry on the stuff. I had to basically force myself to eat something every now and then. I walked into Brian's office weighing well below my typical playing weight.

Apparently, the Giants had struck out on a couple of free-agent first basemen that offseason—their first choices. I was their last resort. It's funny how things work out sometimes. Just when you think you're down and out, God puts an opportunity in front of you that you're not necessarily ecstatic about. Later, you realize it was one of the best things that ever happened to you.

Brian and I talked for 45 minutes about life, baseball, and family. He was very forthcoming and brutally honest, which I absolutely loved. We ended up talking more about my recent Vegas trip than baseball. By the end of the meeting, I was explaining to him how to count cards.

Here I sat, a card-counting, drugged-up hitter in the twilight of his career. Dressed like a rock star. Ego bigger than AT&T Park itself! Chalk this up to another miracle: The Giants signed me.

CHAPTER SIX

INVINCIBLE

"This is why you play. To get an opportunity to play in the playoffs."

—DEREK JETER

Baubi was three months pregnant and starting to show. So many new things to look forward to. Nice two-story townhouse off Clay Street in the Pacific Heights neighborhood of San Francisco. New city. New team. And a new baby boy on the way. Life was great!

I loved going to work again. The air at the stadium had that "new season smell" about it. I knew in my gut that this season was going to be special, and I was so excited to get started. *The Giants have a real shot at being a playoff contender. All the years of getting my ass kicked was sure to end here.* I can't explain why I felt so sure. Maybe it was because of the atmosphere that the entire organization had about it. Not just my teammates, but the front office, maintenance guys, everyone! You could tell everyone here was on board. One big family that truly cared about winning, but more importantly, about each other.

Expectations were high for the entire team, and as one of the new guys in the dugout, I felt like I had something to prove. This would be the first full season I would have with a full wind at my back, Adderall filling my sails. I was excited to see what kind of player I could become.

The season started modestly enough. We were playing decent baseball, and I was hitting for an okay average. Nothing exceptional, but I was holding my own, hitting in spots generally held for the power hitters, fourth or fifth in the lineup, the cleanup spots.

But AT&T Park is basically a hitter's worst nightmare: 421 feet to right center, a 25-foot-high wall. Marine layer. Cold air and wind blowing in off the Pacific. All these elements worked against me to make even my most powerful stroke fall flat.

Standing in the batter's box staring out to right center, that impenetrable fortress of a brick wall seemed a mile away. Hitting it over that wall required way above average power. It makes what Barry Bonds did there, hitting 73 homers in one season, even that much more remarkable. I remember seeing that wall for the first time, feeling like David must have felt facing that other giant, Goliath. It really didn't seem fair that guys who called parks like AT&T home and had to hit half the season in stadiums like this weren't given some sort of handicap. Other guys who called parks like Yankee Stadium home had a distinct advantage. I could easily throw the ball from home plate over the right field wall in Yankee Stadium, and it made no sense to me that the baseball commissioners of the past hadn't thought to standardize park sizes and dimensions, just to even things out a bit. After all, players are paid on stats, so why pay a guy more without consideration of his home venue? The same guy hitting 40 homers in Yankee Stadium would be lucky to hit twenty at a park like AT&T! Seriously. Think about it. Hockey, football, soccer, basketball—all their fields, courts, and pitches are built to the same dimensions. I'm not bitter or complaining, just making an observation. Okay, maybe I am complaining a little bit. Moving on.

The Giants brought me in because I could hit home runs. That was what was expected of me. But two weeks into the season, I still hadn't hit one, not even close. I was growing impatient and frustrated. But probably not as frustrated as the organization or fan base. It was April 14th, and I was sitting on a goose egg. That *had* to change. And soon!

It was an unbelievably beautiful sunny day at AT&T Park. Mind you, almost every day was like that in San Francisco, with temperatures in the mid-60s. There isn't a better place to play a day game in all of major league baseball. I can tell you days were far better than nights, though. During night games, it seemed like the wind conspired with the wall and the dense marine layer to make a batter's life miserable. It blew in from the ocean, bringing with it a damp fog that made it seem impossible to hit anything that even resembled a homer. You could feel the cold, 40-degree wind stabbing you in the face and stinging your eyes as you stepped up to the plate. Day games, however, were a different animal. The direction of the wind magically shifted from the night before, shooing away the marine layer as it blew straight out to center field seemingly winking at you, like it had your back. During the day, you felt like it was possible to get a hold of one, sending it sailing over the wall into the Pacific.

It was my first at bat against Charlie Morton of the Pittsburgh Pirates. I stepped up to the plate, ready to pounce, the usual 20 milligrams doing their thing. I felt confident out there. I dug in and made eye contact, zeroing in on the little one-foot square near his right ear, the little magic square I knew the ball would emerge from.

People ask me all the time, "How do you hit a curveball?" My response is always the same: "Don't miss the fastball!" I knew that if I focused on hitting fastballs, I had a better chance of success. For me, hitting anything off speed was an accident.

My philosophy on hitting has always been to expect a fastball, be ready to crush it, because it may be the only one you get that at bat. I adjusted to anything else. Winged it.

Will "The Thrill" Clark was an idol of mine in my late high school years when he played for the Rangers. The Giants brought him in on occasion to assist with the hitters. I remember him clearly stating his philosophy on hitting to me, "Get the head out, Huffy." He had made a fantastic career out of doing just that, driving the head of the bat through the baseball, racking up an impressive 284 career homers.

When the ball releases from the pitcher's hand and emerges out of that little square space, it could literally be anything. I knew I had roughly 0.40 seconds to determine the pitch type, decide if I was going to swing or let it sail by, finish my stride, get my foot down, and *get the head out*.

For my first pitch, Morton's gift to me was a nice 89-mile-an-hour cut fastball. Even at that rate of speed, the ball seemed to float toward me in slow motion like a big beach ball with a red target on it, almost taunting me, saying, *Hit me into the Pacific.*

Your time to think as a hitter is during batting practice. During a game, you don't have time to think, you simply react. I knew the moment I saw Morton release the ball that I would be unleashing my balanced left-handed stroke. Crack! I felt the power transfer from bat to ball, zero vibration in my hands. The sound when the ball met my 34-inch, thirty-two-ounce, black maple bat was like music to my ears. I dropped my bat and headed toward first base as I watched the trajectory of the ball with delight, knowing I hit it with all I had. *If this ball doesn't go out, I may never hit one here,* I thought. It was a pea-rod rocketing toward the right center field stands. It had the speed and the distance to clear any park in baseball. The crowd stood hushed waiting to see where it would land. I squinted, touching first as the ball was approaching the stands. *Someone in the stands is about to have a souvenir,* I thought. Making my turn for second base, I kept my eyes on the ever-so-shrinking baseball, fully expecting it to sail over the massive wall. The grin quickly disappeared from my face. It was a homer all right, just not the kind I was hoping for.

That impenetrable fortress, my worst enemy, leapt into action. The ball ricocheted hard off the brick archway and rolled in some 90-plus feet toward the right field line where there wasn't a defender in sight.

Adrenaline kicked in as I realized this was my first chance at an inside-the-park homer! I sprinted as hard as I could, lungs bursting out of my chest. Now anyone will tell you that I am not a fast runner, but I felt like I was a cheetah just then. I rounded second, and the crowd went nuts. I locked eyes with third-base coach Tim Flannery. His arms were flailing wildly like those giant windmills I see every time I drive out to Palm Springs. Everything about him, the wild look in his eyes, his posture, shouted RUN! I felt every vein in my neck exerting itself.

Mark DeRosa was hitting next. It was his job to guide me in. I saw him lying face down near home, frantically signaling for me to slide in. *This is going to be close!* As I sprinted toward home, quickly running out of gas, my arms flailed, and I could feel my face turn a beet red. Too tired to try to spot where the ball was by then, I instinctively stuck out my right foot and slid in the last few feet, touching home and righting myself up to end up back on my feet. The roar of the crowd was deafening. I felt vindicated. I just *knew* I had barely snuck this one in. I looked back behind me, and to my dismay, the ball thrown by second baseman Akinori Iwamura was just now reaching the catcher. This wasn't close at all! I was safe by a mile! I gave DeRosa a confused smile. He could tell by looking at my red face that I was about to pass out.

"Sorry, Huffy," he said, trying to stop himself from bursting into laughter. "You have to slide on an inside-the-park homer!" It sure made for a good chuckle for my teammates. A lot of baseball fans say that the inside-the-park home run is the most exciting play in baseball. Well, that may be so, but when you're the guy who hit it, I'd have to disagree.

It was the only inside-the-park homer I had ever (and would ever) hit in my pro ball career, and I would never want to do it again. Homers are supposed to involve a nice leisurely jog around the stadium, breathing in the fresh air, absorbing the fans' adoration, listening to the roar of the crowd as you round third and head home to your welcoming teammates. The only thing that made the run bearable was the Adderall.

A homer is a homer, I guess, and this homer signified a turning point for me. I had broken the goose egg.

Everyone wants to be accepted. Respected. I felt that in spades that season on the field and in the clubhouse. My performance that day gave me the confidence I needed to start hitting with power again. I became the offensive leader the Giants signed me to be.

Off the field was a different story, however. My Adderall use and drinking were out of control. Getting high was all I could think about before I got to the field every day. Immediately after each game, I would retreat to the traveling secretary's office to pull up a comfortable chair, throw back a bucket of ice-cold beers, and suck down a few smokes.

Games wouldn't usually end until around 10 p.m., and by the time I was showered and ready to drive home, it would be around midnight. As if six beers weren't enough, I would always take three more for the ride home! I was living like I was invincible. Like one of those comic book superheroes. I thought I was a badass. In my perverted mind, I felt I deserved the respect and adoration, especially after all the years of losing. This was my time! I was arrogant and had zero respect for what was right or wrong. I didn't feel guilty for any action or behavior. I cared about one person, and one person only. That, my friends, is a scary place to be.

May rolled around, a great time of year to be on the West Coast. I was enjoying the drive to the field one morning, windows rolled down in my black and blue 1969 Mach 1 Mustang, listening to the sound of the 427 Roush racing engine. A far cry from my first car, which I will tell you about later. It was a day game. My phone rang. It was my good friend Pat Burrell. His voice sounded a little heavier than usual. "They just canned me," he said. He went on to explain how he had just been released from the Tampa Bay Rays, and was now, as of an hour ago, a free agent.

Pat and I had always kept in touch, reminiscing over our college days, spit balling about how cool it would be to be teammates once again, especially now we were both big leaguers.

He had enjoyed a great career with the Philadelphia Phillies before signing a free-agent deal with the Tampa Bay Rays. But his union with the organization just wasn't the right fit, and now they had cut him loose with a good chunk of his salary for the Rays to eat. I had played with Pat at the University of Miami. He signed with the Rays three years after I left. I knew back then when he signed that it wouldn't work out well for him with the Rays.

I was a simple, dumb-it-down type of player. "See ball, hit ball." And as luck would have it, that philosophy worked for most of my career. Pat was different. He was a hard-nosed, all-out old-school baseball player. Very professional, and serious in his preparation at the field. He would, on most days, arrive at the field around noon for a game that started at seven, beating the next guy there by two hours. He was meticulous with his video. There wasn't a pitch or a sequence he didn't uncover from each individual pitcher on the opposing team before he took the field for the game that day. He loved and respected the game, and was, and is to this day, truly a student of the game.

The Rays had a different approach than most organizations out there. They were a very small-market franchise, and hardly had any money to sign high-end free agents, let alone keep the talent they had. They had to make do with what they had.

They were a very new-school type of organization, if you will. The exact opposite of Pat's approach. And in baseball, old school and new school never make for a good marriage.

I hung up with Pat, shocked and excited. I pulled into the stadium parking lot with a newfound mission. I knew I had to talk to Bruce Bochy immediately. We had to sign Pat! I just knew he would fit right in with our team of castoffs and misfits.

At the time, we were struggling offensively, and I felt we needed a proven veteran bat in the lineup. Word on the street around that time was that Pat was washed up. But I knew him. And I knew then, as I know now, that given the right supportive environment, any pro can step up to the plate and do his job. I had no doubt that all Pat really needed was a change of scenery and a team that he could truly feel a part of.

Our general manager, Brian Sabean, worked his magic, and on June 4th playing in Pittsburg, Pat and I once again united as teammates. Pat's and my dream became a reality after 12 years as he donned a #9 Giants jersey. And I had a new favorite teammate.

The Giants already had a world-class starting pitching staff in the way of Tim Lincecum, Matt Cain, Jonathan Sanchez, and Barry Zito. We also had a lights-out bullpen rounded out with our eccentric closer, Brian Wilson. The addition of Pat to our lineup reinvigorated us, completing the family. It reinvigorated him, too. He suddenly seemed like he had a new lease on life and fit into the clubhouse very quickly. He and I really fed off each other, almost like my long-lost brother had come back home. With Pat, we started to gel as a team on and off the field.

All the other married men on the team went home to their families after each game. My mind was so invested in the season, I was completely ignoring mine. Even with a pregnant wife and a one-year-old baby boy at home, I spent most of my nights hanging out at bars getting hammered with the locals. It was like I was in college all over again. Most nights I wouldn't stumble back home until three a.m.

San Francisco was not like other cities I had played for. The City by the Bay absolutely worshipped their Giants. People actually recognized you, and I hardly ever had to buy a drink there. The fans fed my ego and encouraged the monster inside me with all the accolades and adoration I craved. It was something new in my experience—actually getting recognized and appreciated for playing baseball. Being treated like a hero. I liked it!

The steady diet of Adderall and beer each night made my already high confidence soar even higher. I absolutely loved the way the people, and especially the young women, of San Francisco would look at me when I walked into a bar. The whole place just stopped and stared. I felt like a rock star every night. Dangerous territory for a married man oblivious to the fact he was in serious danger of losing his family.

August 2010

I don't care how well a team may gel, or how well they have played all year, there always seems to be that one month that doesn't go smoothly. Where key players begin to slump. When worry and doubt begin to creep in. Eventually, that feeling infects the entire team. That month for us happened to be the start of our final-stretch drive.

During August, our ace Tim Lincecum struggled like he had never struggled before, posting a 0-5 record with a 7.82 ERA. He had been our rock at the top of the rotation, and when he began to falter, the fans and the media began to panic, not understanding quite how our 2008 and 2009 Cy Young Award winner could have seemingly lost his stuff. This, in turn, turned up the pressure on everyone who wore a Giants jersey.

The Padres were killing it in the National League West all year. They were sitting comfortably in first place most of the season, and kept pulling away from the pack. We all knew we would have to get really hot, and the Padres had to really cool off if we were going to have *any* chance of catching them.

Our offense began to grip the bats tighter as we tried to hit a home run on every pitch...a recipe for disaster. We were quickly losing our footing in the National League West. If we didn't get this turned around quickly, we were done. We limped into the end of August like a wounded gazelle. The only thing that gave us just the slightest glimmer of hope had nothing to do with us. The Padres were beginning to lose their magic, and a team that had looked unbeatable all season now looked like mere mortals.

Just when we needed to be picking up steam, our team felt like it was starting to falter. I didn't know if we had it in us for the home stretch. We were beat down, and seemingly mentally dead. We needed *something*. A little spark to reignite that passion we had all enjoyed so much earlier that season. So with 30 games remaining, and with an incredibly hard uphill battle in front of us, I decided it was time to bring in a special surprise to the clubhouse to maybe bring us some luck.

AT&T Park was already brimming with the usual media that morning. I walked right past them and my teammates, and marched straight to my locker. A man on a mission. There, I began to strip down out of my street clothes, dropping my jeans to reveal my surprise. A special garment only my wife, Baubi, knew about: A black and red thong with rhinestone letters spelling out PAPI on the front black elastic band, and a skinny red thong running up my crack.

I channeled my inner *Zoolander* and pranced out into the middle of the locker room, right in the middle of the throng of the media, wearing nothing but that black and red Papi thong. Like a battle commander delivering a rally cry, I yelled: "We have 30 more games left, men. When we go 20-10, we will win this division. And this will not come off from under my uniform until we do! Who's with me?"

The media went belly up with laughter. My teammates looked on with...well, I'm not sure if it was disbelief, disgust, amusement, amazement, or maybe a combination of all four.

The media ran with it, of course, writing all about it the next day. Now, I'm not very fond of the media, never have been. I understand that they have a story to write, but I'm not always excited to do interviews.

The rally thong, as it was quickly nicknamed, helped me solve two problems that final month. It helped lift the team's spirits, something we sorely needed, and maybe just as importantly, it helped me avoid pre-game interviews. I would on most days walk around in it for hours in the clubhouse, wearing nothing else. I would read the paper in my black office chair in front of my locker, legs spread wide. And you know what? The media very rarely came within spitting distance of me.

To make things even more unbearable for the poor reporters assigned to the Giants beat, I would walk over to the family-and-friends ticket sign-up sheet right in the middle of the locker room, right where they would be standing, staring, waiting, hoping to talk to someone, anyone, for a snippet to flesh-out into a story. I would watch them all squirm as I bent over with my ass facing directly toward them filling out my ticket request sheet. The guys on the team were about as fond of the media as I was, and this caused them to absolutely lose it every time. Now, don't get me wrong, it wasn't that I had a great body. As a matter of fact, it was quite the opposite. I am a skinny fat guy, if that makes sense. Always have been. Everything looks pretty good with my clothes on, but when I'm naked, it is a complete disaster. My butt cheeks look like I bent over a little too long in the middle of a hailstorm. Hope that gives you a good visual of what I looked like in the thong. You're welcome!

Yep, Aubrey Huff, the small-town, shy kid from Texas was now proudly displaying a red woman's thong in front of some of the most macho athletes in the world. The old Aubrey would never have been caught dead in something like that. Yet now I wore it proudly, like a medal of honor. Adderall is a confidence booster indeed!

September 2010

A new month brings new hope. Baubi was due any day now. I felt energized starting a new month, especially now that I was wearing my secret weapon.

It was September 1st and Tim Lincecum was on the mound for the month's opener against the Colorado Rockies at home. We were confident this was the night Timmy would put his slump behind him. And he did just that, dominating the hard-hitting Colorado offense all night. Timmy was back! And so were we!

The vibe was back and lasted that whole month. The entire pitching staff was untouchable, posting historic numbers for the month of September, going a record 18-straight games giving up three runs or less. The last team to accomplish that feat had been the 1917 Chicago White Sox. We got really hot. And the Padres got really cold, losing 10 games in a row by now. We were right back in this division race, and we couldn't have been more ecstatic. The crowd loved it too, packing the stands each and every game. The electricity and atmosphere were amazing.

On September 10th, we defeated the Padres to finally tie them for first place atop the division. I think we all breathed a collective sigh of relief. We had finally caught them! A feat that seemed impossible that summer. The seven-and-a-half game lead the Padres had on us July 4th was now gone. I have to take my hat off to Timmy. He reinvented himself, shifting his mindset and work ethic from one of a power pitcher to a more balanced, focused machine. He was once again our rock, rallying the team with an impressive September pitching record of 5-1, striking out 52, and only walking six. For the next 15 days, we would trade first place with San Diego. We were not going to make this easy for them. And they were happy to return the favor. The media and the fans were in a feeding frenzy.

I am sure God planned it this way, but early the morning of Wednesday, September 15th, I was actually home and half sober after a 1-0 defeat the previous night by our arch rivals, the Dodgers. Baubi had to knock me out of bed to try to wake me up. Finally, she got my attention with a matter-of-fact tone and said, "Aubrey. It's time. We have to get to the hospital now."

Baubi had the name for our second baby boy picked out well in advance. She is a huge Rolling Stones fan, and there was no arguing or debating what we would call the newest addition to the Huff family. Jagger Ritch Huff it was.

That morning was magical. Seeing the proud look on Jayce's face as he realized he was now a big brother gave me chills. And then seeing my wife hold little baby Jagger made it seem like everything was going to be okay. I felt like the luckiest man in the world holding my baby boy in the rocking chair. I remember thinking, *If I drop dead tomorrow, my life is complete.* In that moment, I had everything I had ever dreamed of as a kid. A beautiful wife; healthy, happy boys; a big league career; and more money than I would ever need. But something else deep down inside of me was tugging at my mind. *I have to get to the field. Now!*

I can only imagine how tired my wife was, not only from the birth, but what I had been putting her through throughout the whole season. Now I was convinced I needed to get to AT&T Park.

In Major League Baseball, you really only get a few opportunities for time off. Funerals and the birth of your child. By league rules, I had three days to spend with Baubi, Jayce, and the new guy on the team, Jagger. But we were headed into the end of the season, and were in the thick of a playoff race. I wasn't about to miss a single game!

First pitch that day was at one p.m. Even though I was running on zero sleep and was still dragging from the game the night before, I knew I had to get back to the stadium. *I'll pop an Adderall and I'll be ready to go*, I thought.

I justified it easily enough. Jagger was born healthy and seemed happy. Baubi was resting peacefully and was in great hands. She had been on bed rest for the final month of the pregnancy, and her mother, Naomi, flew in to be by her daughter's side for that entire month, anxiously awaiting the arrival of her seventh grandchild. *There was not a lot I can do here. I can't help with the feeding. What do I need to be here for?* I reasoned. In fact, I felt that my pacing up and down the corridor, walking around the room like a caged animal, would be more of a nuisance than anything. *Baubi and Jagger need to rest.*

My mind was already made up. I explained to my poor bedbound wife that I was going to play that day. I didn't give her a choice. Off I went, putting baseball ahead of family!

The 10-mile drive from the hospital should have taken 15 minutes. Playing the Dodgers pretty much guaranteed a sellout every time, and today was no different. Don't ask me what these people were doing going to a baseball game midday on a Wednesday. Didn't they have work or school? Either way, it took me an hour to navigate the hordes of fans trying to get to the same place I was headed. I inched along in traffic, sticking out like dog's balls in my car. The only thing moving was the fuel gauge on my Mustang. I finally made it to the field, barely an hour before game time. My teammates looked shocked, as if they couldn't believe I had abandoned my wife in her hour of need. I didn't care. I had to get to my locker. Get my invincible pill, suit up, and get ready for the game.

Every game at this stage of the season is important, but this one seemed even more so. Our division rivals the Los Angeles Dodgers always put up a good fight, determined to beat us up in our own backyard. It was the second game of a three-game series, and good thing I *did* show up. We were up by one in the bottom of the eighth, 1-0. I led off looking to get on base for an insurance run. I hit a double down the left field line. The Dodgers intentionally walked Buster Posey. A wild pitch to Pablo Sandoval let Buster and I move up a bag. I sat there at third, anxious for the next pitch. Sandoval grounded-out to second, and I scored. 2-0.

The Dodgers scored one in the top of the ninth when Andre Ethier hit a solo home run off Brian Wilson. It wasn't enough. 2-1. We won, my run in the eighth inning making all the difference that day. I felt vindicated. Like I had done the right thing by choosing the game over staying with my family.

We had built a three-game lead on the Padres with only three games left in the regular season. And wouldn't you know it, we were to host the Padres for all three games! We only needed to win one out of this three-game set. After nine seasons of defeat, I could literally taste the playoffs.

But with anything in life, the things you want the most seem to be the hardest to get. And in this case it was no different. I thought for sure that we would win one of the first two games. But to our surprise, and to the fans' deafening silence after back-to-back defeats, our lead had all but evaporated, and we were now just one game ahead of our rivals. The final game—our 162nd— was to be played the next day.

I tossed and turned that night, not sleeping a wink. It seemed like none of my teammates did either as we greeted each other the next morning before the big game. The scenario played out like this: If the Padres did, in fact, win, completing an improbable sweep, then we would be at a dead-tie finish for the regular season. We would then have to board a plane that same night and fly to San Diego for a one-game tiebreaker. The winner would be headed to the playoffs. The loser...well, you get the picture.

For a minute, I started thinking maybe I was an albatross around my team's neck. Maybe this would be the closest I would *ever* get to a playoff. I didn't want to find myself in the same position as a season earlier with the Tigers. I love San Diego, but I was in no mood for a trip down there that evening. We *had* to win this game.

Leading up to game time, the clubhouse was eerily quiet. It hadn't felt like that since August. The Padres had some serious momentum and some serious confidence coming in. I can only speak for myself, but I assume many of my Giants teammates feared the worst in the smallest corner of their minds. The game couldn't have started fast enough.

As I took the field to stretch, I had this incredible sense of peace, like I knew everything was going to be okay. The fans all over the stadium had a victorious aura about them as their smiles lit up AT&T. I truly adored the fans there, some of the most passionate on the planet. Then I remembered my promise to my teammates when I had revealed my secret weapon to them a month earlier. Instantly I knew we were going to win this game and send the Padres packing. It was destiny.

It was the bottom of the third when our pitcher Jonathan Sanchez hit a one-out triple. After a strikeout to Andres Torres, Freddy Sanchez stepped up and hit an RBI single up the middle. 1-0. I followed Freddy with a line-drive double to left center, scoring Freddy from first. 2-0. The crowd was going ballistic as I stood there at second triumphant knowing how good our pitchers had been lately. The fat lady was warming up.

A solo home run in the bottom of the eighth by our rookie sensation, Buster Posey, sucked the wind out of the Padres' sails. 3-0.

Top of the ninth, two outs. Our black-bearded closer, Brian Wilson, had two strikes on Will Venable of the Padres. Every seat at AT&T Park was filled, with standing room only beyond the outfield wall. And they were all in full song. Baseball just does not get any more exciting than this.

Baseball involves a lot of standing around, waiting. But I didn't mind standing at first base that day. I remember looking up at the sky before that final pitch, enjoying the rolling white clouds. The finishing touch on a picturesque blue sky. It couldn't have been a more perfect scene as a sea of orange-and-black rally towels waved wildly.

I watched Brian Wilson roll the ball in his glove, positioning it just right. He knew what was at stake. We all knew. It was one of those moments where you are looking around the infield at your teammates. Their eyes telling you everything you already know. I remember looking over at Freddy Sanchez at second, and we smiled at each other. He also had gone his entire career *this close* to the playoffs, never quite making it. The battle was almost over. And I felt it just like my battle-scarred brothers who fought alongside me all year. From spring training, all the way to this very moment, it had indeed been a battle of epic proportions. The anticipation was hard to contain. We all knew that this next pitch could be it.

The windup. The pitch. It was all playing out in slow motion. The ball left Brian's hand at what must have been 93 miles an hour, but it seemed like it was just sailing through the air at the same rate of speed I usually run bases. Strike three!!!

For a split second as the ball sailed past Venable, I heard absolute silence as if the whole world was muted. Then, just as quickly, someone unmuted it, and the sound of victory was absolutely deafening. I don't know what I was yelling at the top of my lungs as I ran to the mound for the celebration. I just know I couldn't hear it above the roar of the crowd.

My prediction of going 20-10 the final 30 days came true. The thong had worked!

At that moment in time, I felt just like I had a month earlier in that hospital room. I felt like everything was okay with the world. My brothers were with me. And for a few moments, time stood still. I was overcome with a complete sense of peace. Like a ton of bricks had just been lifted off my shoulders, allowing me to breathe again. If only my mom, dad, granddad, and my dear grandma who had tossed all those whiffle balls to me as a kid were there in the stands to experience this magical moment with me.

Bruce Bochy encouraged us to take a victory lap, and we did. We jogged around the warning track of the stadium, high-fiving as many fans as we possibly could. I forgot about my real family for a moment. I enjoyed the admiration of the fans and the joy this win brought them, but I struggled to keep it together. My mind took me back to all the disappointing losing seasons, and how I would do it all over again for this brief moment of bliss.

Earlier, I had agreed to a *Baseball Tonight* interview. Now I was kicking myself. I stood there for what seemed like forever in front of the camera, headphones on, waiting for the commercial break to finally be over. I enviously watched every single one of my teammates fire down the dugout toward the clubhouse, ready for their champagne shower.

I can't remember who was about to interview me or what he looked like. I just remember looking at him and mumbling something like, "Sorry, dude, this is taking too damn long. This is my first playoff. I have to get in there with my team and pop champagne." *I had waited long enough in my career for this moment.* And just like that, I tore the headphones off, and I was out of there. I had to be with my brothers.

I felt like a king walking into the locker room. Like one fresh from a battlefield having vanquished his enemy. Like a prodigal son returning home to a welcoming, loving family. I ducked to dodge a champagne cork as it whistled past my right ear. Cold champagne spray rained down on me, drenching my hat and my hair. Stinging my eyes. Dripping into my ears. I reached up, wiping some of it off my face so I could see. It didn't help. The champagne and my tears of joy blended together. I was glad champagne stung. Maybe no one could see my tears.

CHAPTER SEVEN

A TOWN CALLED MARION

*"Winners never quit,
and quitters never win."*

–Vince Lombardi

I was born just north of Columbus, Ohio, in a small town called Marion. I wish I could say I remembered something about my childhood there, but my mom and dad picked up and moved our little family of three to Mineral Wells, Texas, when I was just six months old. I was never told why we moved. I can only assume that my dad had had a rough time making a go of it in the Midwest. Maybe he figured that if he moved closer to family in an oil-rich state, the odds had to be better stacked in his favor.

Mineral Wells was, and still is, a tiny little town. It sits just over an hour west of Fort Worth. It has half the population of Marion, Ohio, and about half as much going on. It's an oil town and used to be a minor tourist attraction with folks coming in from all over the state to enjoy the natural hot springs and wells that gave the town its name.

It feels weird to not know anything about your birthplace, and to not feel any tie to it. Texas would be where I would spend the next 19 years of my life. Outside of a few vacations here and there during my childhood, I never really ventured out of the state. I *feel* Texan because I *grew up* Texan. And even though I live in California now, Texas still has a special place in my heart.

Growing up Texan tends to set one's mind a certain way. Many diehard Texans will tell you there is no reason to ever leave the state; even some of my good friends who live there want to break off into their own republic.

My high school years were different from most of the guys I hung out with; they had a deep Southern toughness about them. They loved to hunt, fish and camp; skills I hadn't been taught. These guys were crazy about their football too, something I couldn't really relate to, likely because not having a dad to throw footballs with defaulted me to my grandparents' favorite sport: baseball.

Texas is a powerhouse football state with deep football pride and tradition that go back generations. If you don't like football, you really don't belong in Texas. At least that's how I felt during my teenage years as I struggled to fit into the typical male stereotype there. I was shy, introverted, awkward, unsure of myself, and not really all that tough. The exact opposite of my high school peers. For the longest time, I felt like I would fit in better in any other state, or country for that matter.

I started high school in Mineral Wells but transferred to a larger school in Fort Worth when my mom landed a better paying teaching job there. I remember her giving my sister and me the option of staying back in Mineral Wells while she commuted the one hour there and one hour back each day, but we all decided as a family to pick up and move. The school in Fort Worth was not that much bigger than the one in Mineral Wells, but they had a better baseball program, and that was all I needed to know.

The new house was about 10 miles from Brewer High School. And I loved the new school the minute I set foot on campus.

Brewer High School in the mid-nineties was a 4A school just west of Fort Worth with about 1200 students, and like every other high school in the state, it enjoyed a very rich football tradition.

High school was a very awkward time for me. Here I was trying to figure out who I was and who my friends were, all while trying to keep my hormones in check. I was desperately trying to fit in, make good grades and focus on baseball. The pressure made me retreat further into my shell. A shell that I had developed following my father's murder when I spent most of my time after school over at my grandparents' house watching the Texas Rangers on television, or painting.

By the time I was nine years old I had grown into quite a baseball fanatic. My mom saw this passion in me, despite the fact I was mediocre at best in my little league efforts. I had developed a passion for art at a fairly young age, and was quite good at it. I was definitely better at painting than at playing ball. In her desperation to connect with her son the way a father would, my mom surprised me after work one day with tickets to go see a Texas Rangers game at Arlington Stadium. I couldn't wait to see the inside of a big league ballpark.

I had just finished an acrylics painting of the Texas Rangers logo on a canvas just a few weeks earlier and brought it along in hopes of scoring autographs from some of my favorite players. I raced through the gates of the stadium immediately trying to find my way toward the home dugout where I was sure I would get lucky. My mom and sister tried desperately to keep up. Batting practice had just begun. I was awestruck by the size of the Rangers players as they walked by me, and by the confidence they exuded. It was intoxicating. I had no idea what a man was, but after one look at these guys, I knew this was the kind of man I wanted to be. I scored thirteen autographs from some of my favorite Rangers that day. I was in heaven!

I walked out of that stadium proudly carrying that painting above my head, feeling like I were ten feet tall. It still hangs on my man room wall today and marks the day I knew beyond a shadow of doubt what I wanted to be. I couldn't tell you who won the game that night, but I can still smell the stadium and hear the sounds that can only be experienced in person at a game.

I was anything but tired as my mom buckled my sleepy sister in the back seat of the car. We hadn't even left the parking lot for the hour and fifteen-minute drive back to Mineral Wells when I hit her with it.

"Mom, I know what I want to be when I grow up. A Major League Baseball player."

She responded as you can imagine most moms would, "That's nice sweetheart." That response simply wasn't good enough for me. I continued excitedly, "Mom, if you buy me a batting cage and a pitching machine I promise you I'll buy you a house and a car one day!" Her response wasn't what I was hoping for, "Baby you know I would in a second if I had the money. Maybe someday."

That someday came just months later, but it may as well have been years for me. I hounded my poor mother every day for the next five months about that cage. Then, on December 15th, just five days before my 10th birthday, my mom led me out to our half-acre backyard, her hard-working calloused hands covering my eyes while she guided me over the deck, down the steps and toward the back fence. *Is it what I think it is?* I thought to myself in giddy anticipation. Sure enough! I opened my eyes.

"Surprise! Happy Birthday! And Merry Christmas!"

There it was. A 65-foot long, 15-foot-wide batting cage, Jugs pitching machine, and a 20-ball automatic feeder. It was all I would get for my birthday and for Christmas that year. It would have been just fine for me if that was all I got for the next 10 years! It was everything I had envisioned. I hugged my mom as hard as I could, and raced over to the cage. I didn't have a bat with me, but I didn't care! I just wanted to be in it!

I sat down inside the cage, leaning my back up against one of the pitching machine legs, eyes wide, mind racing. It was clear what I needed to do to achieve my dream. I made up my mind right there and then that I wouldn't sleep until I hit at least 200 balls a day. And that's what I did.

From that day until I graduated from high school, I hit 200 balls a day. Sometimes 300. With every swing, I envisioned myself hitting a home run in a big World Series game. Right down the right field line at Arlington Stadium, the only stadium I had ever set foot in. That is until my junior year in 1994 when the Rangers moved into a newer field, The Ballpark in Arlington. The same ballpark my vision would become reality in some 16 years later.

Most guys in high school are thinking about girls and football growing up. Not me. The only thing on my mind was baseball. But regardless of how much time I spent in the batting cage, hitting baseball after baseball, I wasn't seeing any results in any of the games. I had a nice swing, actually a beautiful swing, but it just wasn't yielding the kind of results I expected of myself. It wasn't like I was slacking off playing video games. I was working hard, hitting a ton of balls, doing all I knew to improve, with no noticeable effect. It was pretty demoralizing.

Yep, my high school career as a Brewer Bear was pretty dismal. I hit right around .300 and hit just one home run my entire varsity career. Not exactly the type of production you would expect out of a future big leaguer. I was a lanky, awkward kid. I had already hit six feet four inches, and had just 180 pounds on my frame. Like a newborn giraffe trying to find its legs, I had little to no coordination. I was passionate about the game of baseball, but passion was not enough. There is no nice way to say it. I just wasn't all that good at baseball in high school. Where I did find success, however, was in basketball. My mom had something to do with that.

My mom was an excellent basketball player during her high school days in Haskell, Texas, a very small farming community near Abilene with a population of maybe 1000. She always liked to brag to me that she had scored 50 points in a game once. I didn't think much of this when I was younger, but I think that's a pretty impressive feat for *any* player at *any* level. I loved my mom. I know that sounds like a given, but I wasn't one of those smart-aleck kids who took his parents or grandparents for granted, or thought of them as a hassle or headache to deal with. I truly appreciated how hard my mom worked to provide the best she could for my sister and me. I pounced on any opportunity I could to connect with her, and basketball was definitely a language she understood.

I remember one day in particular in the late spring of 1986 when I was 10. My mom burst through our front door after work, still in her work clothes, and with her usual sweet smile said, "Aubrey, come outside with me. Let's shoot some hoops."

I jumped at the chance. I knew nothing about the game, other than what I learned from watching it on TV, but I figured hey, it's a chance to spend time with my mom, doing something she loves. We headed outside to our driveway to a cheap, tattered basketball hoop she had set up long ago in hopes I would take to the game, but I never really had the interest. The hoop was missing the net, and looked like it could keel over at any minute, but it didn't matter. Those 45 minutes hanging out with my mom having fun felt like we were in an NBA arena.

Over the course of a few months, my mom worked with me an hour or two each night, four nights a week, teaching me everything she knew about basketball. I find myself tearing up even now, remembering my sweet mom shooting three-pointers with me in her Winn-Dixie uniform, sweat on her brow, the biggest smile on her face. That love and dedication she had for my sister and me still amazes me to this day. It didn't matter how exhausted she was, she always seemed to find a little in the reserve tank to play one-on-one with me, or sit and read with my little sister.

Now that I have had 30 years to reflect, I guess playing basketball with me did not seem like a chore to her, more like an escape from reality. A chance to be a kid again and have some fun. Like all parents, she was looking for a connection with her child. Something she could teach me, to pass knowledge down to me. She couldn't teach me to hunt or fish. I could tell she was excited to have finally found a connection. Basketball wasn't my favorite sport, but seeing the love my mom had for it made me respect it.

I made the school basketball team and quickly found my place. The stuff my mom had shown me—trick shots, dribbling techniques, using my body to block out the other guy to get in position for a rebound, and general ball awareness to make my way down the court all paid off. I was named MVP of the team in each of my two varsity seasons. I played power forward, and was the type of player who could handle the basketball well and slam dunk when I had an open breakaway. But my best trait was the ability to shoot. Again, I give credit to my mom for working with me on how to just perfectly launch the ball regardless of my rate of speed or travel direction. I was a pretty decent three-point shooter. Even so, I certainly did not fool myself into thinking I could ever be anything more than a good *high school* player.

Basketball was fun, but baseball was my passion. Because of that, I never really felt I was a star at basketball. It came too easily for me, if that makes sense. When things come so easily, it's hard to feel like you deserve success. My heart simply wasn't in it. But I have to be honest, I was way better at basketball at that particular time of my life than baseball.

Ask anyone who's survived high school and they will tell you that one year in particular stands out more than any other: senior year. It's the last year you'll ever *have* to go to school. It's also the time most finally start thinking about moving away from home to start a life as an adult. It's a dramatic transition. My senior year was a very confusing time. I had absolutely no idea what I was going to do next. My dream was to earn a scholarship to some big Texas college like Texas Tech, Texas A&M, UT, or TCU, but I soon realized that I just didn't have the statistics I needed for a chance with any of those schools. My high school baseball career was pretty unimpressive. I felt my Major League Baseball dream slipping through my fingers and this caused me a great deal of anxiety. Baseball was my Plan A. It always had been. I didn't have a Plan B or C. There's not much worse than that moment in life when you realize that you don't have what it takes, having your Plan A deflated and your dreams evaporate before your eyes.

I walked around campus in an almost zombie-like state for a few weeks. Everyone around me seemed to know exactly what their plans were. Some were excited about colleges they had committed to. Others had decided to be done with school, and were happy with that. Everyone seemed to be making plans for the future, except for me. I know I wasn't the only one in that boat, one without a rudder, but it sure felt like it at the time. I finally accepted the fact that sports would not play a part in my future. I knew I had to come up with a Plan B, and quick.

It's funny how as soon as you give up on something, God seems to throw you a bone to keep your spirits up, your hopes alive. To my surprise, I came home one day to find a letter in the mail from a small Division 2 school in Kansas, inviting me to be a part of its basketball team. I was floored. By this time I was done mourning my baseball career that would never be. I had already given up on baseball, and I certainly wasn't expecting anything from basketball. As a young kid I was a dreamer, but high school had quickly made a realist out of me. I was a slow, six-four white dude who could barely dunk. I am not sure what the guys from Kansas saw in me, but apparently they saw enough to offer me a small scholarship. I had some serious thinking to do.

I knew beyond a shadow of a doubt that if I chose college basketball, that's where my athletic career would end. There was no way I would ever become an NBA player. Again, I didn't love basketball; I loved baseball.

The fork in the road had finally arrived. The road to the left led to Kansas. The one to the right led to skipping the whole college experience altogether. I would grow up, get a job in the fast-food industry, and stop dreaming about the major leagues. Graduation was just around the corner, and I couldn't push the thought out of my head that I was a failure. I felt melancholy at best. I struggled to accept a future that saw me never leaving Texas, marrying the first woman who came along, and having eight kids. I knew what was coming, a balding head and a beer gut to show off at my 20-year high school reunion, where I would talk about the glory days. That was a vision I had a hard time swallowing.

I tossed and turned at night, struggling with the pressure of having to choose between chasing a dream and giving up on life.

The harder I tried to come up with a Plan B, the more trouble I had truly letting go of baseball. One night, in the dead of night, I awoke from a deep sleep and sat straight up in bed. *I have to give my baseball dream another chance,* I determined. *I have worked so hard in that cage. So many years of hard work! I owe it to myself!*

As luck would have it, I heard about an open tryout at a small junior college three hours northwest of Fort Worth. Then called Vernon Regional Junior College, the two-year community college had a small baseball program. Jay Arnold and Jason Keathley, my high school teammates, decided to try out and invited me to tag along. This was the chance I was looking for. I remember thinking of this fork in the road like a coin toss. *If I make the team, I will play for the Vernon Chaparrals. If not, I will take the Kansas basketball scholarship and see where that leads.* Heads, Vernon; tails, Kansas. Easy choice. Or so I thought.

Tryout day came and the three amigos set sail to Vernon. I felt like I gave it my all that morning, fielding ground balls by no means smoothly, but decently enough. My hitting was way worse. Every time I made contact with the ball it felt like I was swinging with a wet newspaper. I simply had zero power. A 6 foot 4 inch 185 pound slap hitter. Everything seemed like a struggle, and I walked away feeling pretty disappointed and embarrassed with my performance, knowing full well I had made a huge mistake by trying out.

The head coach of the Chaparrals, Danny Watkins, must have seen something in my swing though as he decided miraculously to give me a shot. All three of us got called back in fact. Even though I didn't have a scholarship, it worked financially for my mom. Vernon was a small, inexpensive school. It was a safe choice, too, since it was just a three-hour drive to Mineral Wells if I decided to come home for the weekends. And so the coin landed. Heads! Vernon!

I remember thinking, *You have a second shot at this. Don't blow it.* I stood in front of the mirror in my new dorm bathroom. I had to figure out how to get better. I had already tried everything I knew to better myself in high school, working endlessly in my cage. But that wasn't cutting it. *What can I do?* I asked myself.

I stood staring at a tall skinny awkward boy in the mirror. I knew I had to get bigger and stronger, fast. A nice left handed swing alone just wasn't going to cut it if I were to advance from a junior college team. I had to stand out. I had to begin hitting with more power.

With three short months before my debut as a Chaparral, I committed to working out twice a day and practicing twice as long as everyone else. I ate like a machine, going in for seconds, sometimes even thirds. I had a dream. Now it was time to start grinding to make that dream a reality.

The camaraderie our team of 25 guys shared in that baseball dorm was amazing. I still indulged in having a few pops with the fellas on the team every so often, but for the next 12 weeks, I was focused on one thing and one thing only: a Division 1 Texas scholarship somewhere. I had a plan to play out my two seasons as a Chaparral, earning a full scholarship on a team at a bigger university. I was a man on a mission. I wasn't going to blow this chance. Nothing was going to stop me. I was going to will this to happen.

My new schedule saw me waking up every morning ready to hit the gym and lift weights at six a.m. I would follow that with a massive breakfast, class, and finally baseball practice. This is where the rest of my teammates called it a day, but not me. After every player had left practice, I would go into the cage and hit solo for an hour or more. By then, I would be starving, so I would eat a hefty dinner. Then I would work out for the second time, often not stopping until well into the evening. I collapsed into bed every night exhausted, only to wake up at six a.m. and do it all over again. The only break from this routine came on Saturday nights when I hung out with my teammates.

Spring came. The first game as a Chaparral was here. I looked and felt like a different person. I looked like the boy in me had been shed, revealing a real man underneath. I felt like a man too. I had transformed my six-foot-four-inch frame from 180 pounds of weakling to 220 pounds of lean muscle. I was in the best shape of my life. Opposing pitchers didn't stand a chance.

That first season at Vernon was like child's play. From the first game to the last, I felt like I was playing on another level, like I wasn't supposed to even be there. I had never had so much confidence on the baseball field, and it translated into my stats. The one single home run during high school became a distant memory as I knocked it out of the park, literally, with seventeen home runs. I had always had the nice swing, but now with the added strength that my new routine had produced, my nice swing translated into a force to be reckoned with.

That newfound level of confidence translated into real results for me that season. I was unanimously voted as the team MVP and was able to secure a spot on the all-regional team for our conference. I could barely believe any of this was happening! I was so happy that I had made the decision to pursue my dream. *Just one more year grinding it at Vernon and I'll be off to a major university,* I thought. The dream was clear again. I was having fun and another year seemed like it would fly by. Sometimes, however, plans work out way quicker than you expect.

CHAPTER EIGHT

REDNECK AT A COUNTRY CLUB

"Everything you want
is on the other side of fear."

—Jack Canfield

May, 1996.

With the year at Vernon officially over, I got busy packing my dorm room in preparation for summer back in Fort Worth. I was nursing a major hangover, cramming my belongings into boxes, when I heard a knock on my door.

"Huffy, phone call," one of my teammates announced. There was one payphone in the dorm for all 25 guys to share and apparently someone was on the line waiting for me. *Mom,* I thought. I headed to the lounge section and picked up the phone to an unfamiliar male voice with a deep Southern accent.

"Hey big guy, this is Turtle Thomas, hitting coach for the University of Miami Hurricanes. You want to fly out to Miami for a tryout?" Talk about right to the point!

My first instinct was doubt. In our dorms, we had a very funny group of guys who loved to play pranks, and I was convinced this was one of those tricks. *No way would a powerhouse baseball program like the Miami Hurricanes be interested in me,* I thought. "Ha ha! Very funny guys, but you're not getting me." I hung up.

I got word that Coach Watkins wanted to see me later that day before I took off for home. So after loading my truck and saying bye to my teammates, I stopped by his office. I had barely closed the door behind me when coach spit out his dip and yelled excitedly, "Damn, Aubrey! What's your problem?"

I was confused. "What do you mean?" I replied.

"How can you hang up the phone on Turtle Thomas when I put so much work into getting Miami to look at you?"

My heart sank. I felt the blood drain out of my head and almost threw up right then and there. I explained how I thought I was being pranked, and after a good belly laugh, Coach Watkins told me that even after all that, they still wanted me to fly out for a tryout. "Are you interested?" he asked.

I will never forget Coach Watkins' unending belief in me, even when I didn't believe in myself. He put his reputation on the line to get me in front of one of the most prestigious baseball schools in the country. I must have said thank you 20 times before he finally shook my hand and kicked me out of his office.

With the Vernon campus disappearing in my truck mirrors, I knew without a doubt that this would be the last time that I would lay eyes on it. Part of me was sad. Sad that I didn't have a chance to say a proper good-bye to my newfound brothers. Funny how baseball works. You are literally family for half a year. You go through the blood sweat and tears together. Then in a flash, it's over. And you never see each other again.

Two weekends later I took batting practice at Mark Light Stadium, home of the Miami Hurricanes with six or seven other prospects. I was far from home, but confident and excited for the opportunity. My tryout went as expected. I fielded ground balls at first base flawlessly, and my batting practice was a power display from foul pole to foul pole. I could get a sense from the coaches that they were definitely interested in me. I walked away fully convinced I had performed far better than any of the other guys. I started envisioning myself on this same field a few months into the future, holding my own against some of the best players in the country.

The Hurricanes had lost the College World Series the previous year to Louisiana State University on a bottom-of-the-ninth-inning walk-off home run. No doubt the most heartbreaking loss you could ever suffer in a baseball game. I was sure they would be hungry to get back to Omaha to play for the national championship on ESPN, and I desperately wanted to be a part of that. I walked away confident I had made the cut, but my nerves almost got the better of me over the next week hanging out at my mom's house in Fort Worth.

After hanging up on Henry "Turtle" Thomas back at the dorm, there was no way I was going to miss a call from the University of Miami. I was afraid to even go to the bathroom that whole week. I sat by the phone waiting for it to ring, picking it up and checking for a dial tone every hour or so, like some high school kid anxiously waiting for *the* call from the hot girl in school. A few days passed, and even though the coaches at the tryouts had clearly told us it would be a week or so before any decisions were made, I started doubting myself. *Had I given them the right phone number?* I asked myself. *What if they were trying to call me back at the dorm?* Finally, after one of the longest weeks of my life, the call came.

My heart was racing a million miles an hour as I picked up the receiver.

"Hey big guy, you want to be a Miami Hurricane?" It was Turtle Thomas. Without hesitation I said, "Absolutely, big guy." From the minute I met Turtle, I knew he was going to be a tremendous influence in my baseball career. Turtle was the kind of guy that knew how to motivate you. He's a no-nonsense type coach who knows how to push just the right buttons to get you to play the way you're capable of playing. If you wanted extra work, then he was your guy. He was always the first one to the field and the last one to leave. Not only was he one of my all-time favorite coaches, he is now still to this day one of my good friends.

We spoke for 20 minutes about the history of the program, what was expected of me, and, of course, my scholarship. He told me that the school was only willing to take care of half of my tuition, but increasing it to a three quarter scholarship for the next year. Miami is a pretty expensive school, and even with half of my tuition in scholarship, it was going to be a stretch for my mom, but she knew how big of an opportunity this was for me, and once again, she was there backing me up 100 percent, sacrificing every luxury to give me a shot at a real future.

The big day finally came. I would be taking my boots, my flannels, my Southern drawl, and my trusty 1988 extended-cab Chevy pickup truck to the vibrant streets of Miami, Florida. I was going to fit in like a redneck at a country club.

I was excited about the chance to play for the Hurricanes, but that little voice inside my head was stuck on replay. *You're not going to last a week down there, Aubrey.*

The drive from Texas to Miami was scary as hell for me. Here I was in my rusty red truck with 90,000 miles on it, barreling down I-20 at 75 miles an hour into uncertainty. Well, uncertainty is the wrong word. I was certain of one thing: failure.

Thoughts of rejection danced in my head. How the hell was a small-town kid like me going to fit into the loud, obnoxious culture of Miami? *How will I get along with some of the best players in the country at a real powerhouse program? Am I going to be good enough to cut it?*

I had a lot of time to wrestle with my thoughts on that long drive. As one of the premier baseball schools in the country, Miami was expected to make it to the College World Series in Omaha, Nebraska each and every year. Anything short of that was considered unacceptable, a massive failure. With these high expectations came an even higher standard for each of the players on the team.

Everything was happening so fast. *Was last season a fluke? How can I be sure I'm really good enough to play for the Hurricanes?* After all, I had been a below-average high school player, then seemingly out of nowhere I was a superstar in junior college. *But Division 1 baseball is a whole new ballgame.*

This would be the first time I would be away from home for any real amount of time. *What if anything goes wrong? Or what if I just want to come home for the weekend?* Sixteen hundred miles one way is not exactly a quick weekend trip. My time in Vernon was pretty safe. I drove home every other weekend to visit my mom and hang with high school buddies. My mom was my best friend at that time of my life. You could even say I was a big time mama's boy. Now, that safety net, the ability to go home any time, was quickly disappearing in my rattling rearview mirror. I crossed the Texas-Louisiana border.

As I glinted into the early morning sun, a weird sensation washed over me. Even without air conditioning, it wasn't hot in the cabin, but I was sweating. My palms were clammy as I gripped the wheel at 10 and two. I could see my knuckles turn white as my grip tightened, and with it, my chest. My breathing grew shallower. I felt my heart beat harder than normal. I started to see everything in weird colors, like everything was being processed through an Instagram filter.

What the hell is happening here? I thought to myself. Then I realized—it hit me like a Mack truck—I wasn't a kid anymore. I was officially on my own. I didn't have my mommy anymore. It was time to become a man. I wasn't sure if I knew how to be one.

Any energy I had drained out of me.

I crossed into Mississippi tired and hungry. I could have curled up and taken an eight-hour nap right there, but I knew I still had 800 miles ahead of me, so I grabbed some gas and a burger, and drove on to Mobile, Alabama. I crashed there for the night.

It was a weird night's sleep. I slept, but I did not feel rested. My body went to sleep, but my mind didn't, instead it engaged in warfare all night over the uncertainty of my future. At this time of my life, I hated change. I liked knowing what each day was going to bring. Being back home in Texas where I wasn't entertaining all these negative thoughts sure sounded like a more comfortable place to be. More comfortable than that Motel 6, that's for sure.

As I drove deeper east into the Florida Panhandle with the windows rolled down, it felt like someone had flipped the scenery switch on me. *We're not in Texas anymore,* I thought. Everything looked and smelled different. Palm trees rocked gently in the breeze as far as the eye could see. The sight and smell of the ocean calmed my nerves if only for a few minutes. I passed a sign welcoming me to Miami. I started to get excited again.

I had never seen so much traffic and diversity. My two days trying out for the Hurricanes a few months prior were a whirlwind. I was on a two-day mission to make the team and had no time for distractions or to take in the environment around me. Now, I soaked it in.

In Texas you try to draw as little attention to yourself as possible. You wear earth-tone-colored flannel shirts, relaxed-fit Levi's jeans, and a pair of dirty work boots as you go about your day with a quiet, respectful, hardworking confidence. Miami seemed to be the complete opposite. It was loud, and the people seemed very disrespectful. There was a sense of entitlement there that I had never felt in all my life. My deep-seated Texas roots were about to get culture-shocked. I knew right then I would be completely out of my element.

Turtle had arranged for me to share an apartment with two seniors on the team for the first year so they could show me the ropes. I was really looking forward to meeting my new roommates, especially after the amazing experience I had just had with my old family at Vernon. Turtle told me one of the guys would be there to let me in.

The apartment complex was a quick 15-minute drive from campus, and I had no trouble finding it. I pulled into the first parking spot I could find and got out. After what seemed like weeks on the road, it felt so good to finally get out and straighten my legs. The hot sun on my face reminded me of a hot Texas day. But it was a different heat there. The humidity was almost unbearable. *This is going to take some getting used to*, I thought.

I knocked excitedly on the apartment door. I stood there like an idiot for what seemed like five minutes waiting for someone to come to the door, wondering if I had the right apartment.

Finally, the door swung open. I was met by Ryan Grimmet, a senior who played center field, and another senior, Kevin Nykoluk, the team catcher. My new roommates. *Douchebags*. I knew it the minute I laid eyes on them.

My excitement to meet these two men turned into disgust within a week of rooming with them. I had never been around such egotistical, unhelpful, rude individuals in all my life. Not only did they give me a hard time 24/7, but they never even offered me the courtesy of the basics: showing me around town and introducing me to any other guys. Guys would come over to hang out regularly, yet Ryan and Kevin never even acknowledged my existence, let alone introduce me to any of them, or ask me to go anywhere with them. It seemed like I was an outcast before I even moved in.

I was already reaching for the rip cord three days in, ready to bail out of that hellhole of an apartment. But what choice did I have? I couldn't call Turtle crying. I had to suck it up! *Surely this will get better once I get to know these guys better.*

All the abuse I was taking at the apartment made me look forward to the very first fall practice with my new team even more. I figured the rest of the guys on the team couldn't be as bad as the two jerks I was living with.

I would be wrong.

Nervous excitement struck again as I stepped into the locker room at Mark Light Stadium for the first time. I was really looking forward to meeting all my new teammates and coaches, happily anticipating a brand new year of doing what I loved: playing ball.

Even as I write this so many years later, I still remember what it felt like walking in. The atmosphere in that locker room just exuded confidence, and I immediately felt like a small fish in a big pond. Like a tee-ball kid walking into the dugout of his favorite pro team with a poster in hand, looking for autographs. I must have been the only guy in there who was absolutely terrified. Everyone else appeared to have it all together and looked and acted like they belonged there. I had never seen so many guys who actually *looked* like baseball players. Every single guy I was introduced to looked like they could play in the big leagues right then and there. And one guy in particular stood out more than any other. Pat Burrell.

Pat was a sophomore and the alpha male of the entire team. He had just become the first freshman in Miami history to win the NCAA batting title the year prior. He was a hitting machine and already looked like—and carried himself like—a big leaguer. At six feet five inches, 225 pounds with broad shoulders, square jaw, and rugged good looks, he was what I like to call a man-child.

I would always catch the ladies at the University of Miami tripping over themselves anytime they passed by Pat on the way to class. And you could hardly blame them. There was just something different about this guy. The way he owned the room. It was as if he *knew* he was going to be in the big leagues one day.

Pat was everything I was not: he had a relaxed confidence, a natural leadership ability, and a witty sense of humor. Nothing seemed to bother him, he would just glide through a room, with chin up, shoulders back, chest out, and a bit of a strut that told everyone in that locker room he was the head lion. And it seemed like every single guy in that locker room worshipped him.

I thought to myself, *How can someone be that confident? Was he born like that? Did he learn it from his father?* I watched his every move, trying to imitate not so much his swing, but the way he carried himself. In all my life I had never met a guy who displayed so much masculinity. I desperately wanted to be like that.

Now that I am a father myself, I am absolutely convinced that it is impossible for a boy to grow into a strong confident man without a father or close male figure showing him how. Without a father, you can't really escape that feeling of incompletion. You can never get rid of that longing for confidence, strength, adventure and danger. You can never fill that hole deep in your heart.

It took me a long time to fill that hole. To shake that feeling I desperately craved so that I wouldn't be terrified deep down in my soul, beneath that brave, tough exterior. That constant worry and anxiety that I just didn't measure up in this world. To my wife. My children. My career.

In the movie *Fight Club*, Ed Norton plays a man who is fed up with the monotony of life. He works in a job that he absolutely hates. He has no woman to go home to. Instead, he sits in his quiet, quaint little apartment, furnished with trendy IKEA furniture. His refrigerator is empty except for condiments. A crippling case of insomnia haunts him. He hates who he has become as a man.

Norton's character (who is never given a name) is desperately trying to fit into the mold that society has burned into his brain. What society tells him a real man is supposed to be. His laugh oozes with depression and has a sick sadness about it. As he is flying across the country to yet another meeting one day, he secretly wishes the plane would crash so that he could be put out of his misery. This is when he conjures up his alter ego, Tyler Durden, played by Brad Pitt. Tyler is everything he is not. Handsome, confident, brash, fearless, and free. He absolutely hates authority, and all the rules society tries to bind him with. He becomes his alter ego Tyler Durden, so that he no longer has to deal with who he really is inside. I can relate.

I lived like that for 20 years. Turning myself into something I'm not because I didn't know how to be a real man. I got frosted tip highlights in my hair. I sat in countless tattoo parlors, getting inked all over my body because I thought that would make me look tougher than I actually was. I even had the Transformers Autobot and Decepticon insignia tattooed on my shoulder blades and would constantly wear my hat backward like a teenager as if to say, *Hey, I am kind of a badass, but I don't want to be taken too seriously.* I trapped the real me deep down inside with endless nights of booze and drugs just so I could keep him dormant.

I didn't like the real me. The real me was a pansy. I wanted to be a real man but didn't know how. And I wasn't desperate enough to create my own alter ego. Yet.

Once fall baseball practices at the U got into full swing I quickly became the resident punching bag. I wasn't sure what everyone's deal was, but for some reason every guy on the team was ripping on my clothes, my accent, my virginity...

At this time in my life, I was just like any other college male. Hormones were at an all-time high. I was just a simple guy from Texas, always respectful of women. I wanted to wait until marriage because I believed it was the right thing to do, and it was the way my mom had raised me. Plus, it kept me focused on my game.

In Texas there were guys I knew in high school and college who were having sex. But it wasn't really talked about all that much. Bragging about it was considered rude and demeaning to the girls. Quite frankly, it was just assumed that it was nobody else's business.

Here, women were just a sport. It seemed like half of our conversations at the University of Miami were about sex. These guys talked more about women than about baseball; it was weird. When the team found out I was a virgin, it was all over but the crying for me.

The pounding never ended. It started when I stepped into the locker room each day. The first thing someone would yell was "Hey it's time for the Aubrey Huff virginity update." I wanted the floor to open up and swallow me. To say it was embarrassing would be a gross understatement. I'd be red in the face from embarrassment one minute, and from absolute rage the next. I was ready to explode and wanted to beat the hell out of every dude on that team. But I wasn't the confrontational type. I had zero balls and was scared to death to defend myself. These guys acted worse than high school kids with a few too many beers in them.

The absolute worst part of each day by far for me was team stretch. Apparently it was a big tradition to circle up as a team down the right field line at Mark Light Stadium and unleash a series of scathing verbal attacks on one another. Nothing was out of bounds. From rude comments about your family or girlfriend, to insults about the size of your johnson or lack thereof. The amount of trash talking I experienced there is something I have yet to ever experience again. I've never seen such hostility toward human beings, not to mention teammates.

I was the brunt of those attacks on most days. Sounds like I am making it up, but that 10 minutes of stretch felt like ten years of hell for me. I absolutely hated it and found it all pretty confusing. I had no idea why everyone had such hostility toward me. I was a pretty quiet guy...barely ever said a word. I was just trying to fit in and be as nice as I possibly could to everyone. Being nice got me nowhere. All I got in return were insults and degrading remarks, as if they were pushing me to the breaking point for fun. I wouldn't wish that kind of punishment on my worst enemy.

I wasn't much for snappy comebacks. I had never had the need because I had never been around such disrespectful pricks in my life. Instead of retaliating with one-liners when my teammates were hurling abuse, I just stuffed it all in and gave them all an uncomfortable smile while doing my stretching. Inside, I was on the verge of either tears or ripping someone's head off. A ticking time bomb.

It really sucks when you're the joke and you're not even in on it. I was just so serious that I didn't see the sarcasm or the fun in any of it until much later. It didn't dawn on me until later that year that this was just a form of hazing. It was all just a test to see if I had what it takes to play for the Miami Hurricanes, and if I could mentally handle the pressure that was sure to come during the baseball season. And everyone was in on it. Even my roommates Ryan and Kevin. I realized then that they weren't douchebags. They were just all trying to mentally toughen me up for not only baseball, but life. And in a weird way I was thankful for that lesson.

I am here to admit that I became the same kind of jerk. I really feel bad for some of the abuse I hurled at rookies as I got older, but at the same time I knew it would help them toughen up or they would be gone. It was a great weeding-out process. Either you can handle it and stay, or you weren't mentally strong enough and had to go back home. Baseball is a game for the absolute strongest of mental fortitudes. If you're not strong mentally, you're as good as dead.

When I was on the receiving end of all this abuse, I dealt with it all the only way I knew how. I isolated myself from everyone. All I did every day was go from school, to practice, to my apartment. There, I would lock my bedroom door and watch TV, sometimes crying myself to sleep. I was ready to get out of the apartment. Out of Miami. I was just waiting for the final straw so I could fly back home to Texas.

My baseball game that first month suffered immensely. I don't care how much athletic or natural ability you have, unless you're happy, you can't succeed. That's true for baseball, and more importantly for life.

I hear people say all the time, "Once I become successful, then I'll be happy." It took me a while to figure this out, but I am convinced that you have to be happy, otherwise you will never be successful. You can't have one without the other. I was definitely not happy. And I was definitely not going to be successful on the field under these conditions.

The straw that broke the camel's back came one typical muggy Miami morning. I was about two months into my new-found hell, circling the campus lot like an idiot, trying to find a parking spot. Parking there was a nightmare. The spaces were barely big enough for a Volkswagen bug, let alone a regular size car. Now keep in mind, my red 1988 extended cab Chevy truck was longer, taller, wider, and harder to navigate than anything else on the road down there. That truck was a nightmare to drive and even harder to park.

I explored every inch of the campus lot and side streets for 20 minutes. Not a single spot was to be had. I was getting really annoyed. Then, just like a mirage in the desert, I spotted an opening about 20 spaces ahead to the right. I could see another dude headed in that direction, but he was in the next row. He'd been doing the same dance I had, and probably felt just as annoyed and desperate as I was at that point. I hit the gas, and with a puff of gray smoke I hustled over to the spot with my turn signal blinking, like a dog marking his territory. There was a small Toyota pickup truck parked right on the line on the left side, and a Jeep on the other. It was going to be tight, but at this point I was already late for first period and had to try to maneuver into it. I full-locked the wheel and crawled in at a mile an hour. "Damn!" I'd hit the car to my left making it rock a little in place. The sickening sound of good old American chrome (albeit a little rusty) tearing into Japanese plastic made me cringe. I started backing out so I could get a better angle on the spot. A different sound of metal crunching rang in my ears. *You gotta be kiddin' me!* I'd hit the car parked behind me.

My truck was as out of its element as I was on campus. This was the sign I was looking for. I don't think it could have been any clearer if there was a neon sign flashing "Aubrey, what are you doing? You don't belong here, go back home to Texas!"

I was defeated. I was frustrated and embarrassed. *To hell with this, I am headed back to Texas,* I thought. *Who was I kidding? I'll never make it out here!*

CHAPTER NINE
THE U

"Arrogance is the camouflage of insecurity."

—Tim Fargo

I pulled out of that parking lot, tail between my legs, pushing any thoughts of going to class out of my head. I had my mind set. *I'm getting out of Miami.*

The drive back to the apartment was an emotional one. What welcomed me when I got there sealed the deal. The first words out of Kevin's mouth were, "Hey, virgin, get me a water while you're up, will ya?" I shuffled to the fridge, almost like I was his own personal butler, tossed a bottle of water in his direction, and retreated to my room feeling beat down and worthless.

I closed the door behind me and dug into a bowl of M&M's, trying hard not to cry, pushing away the thoughts of failure that were plaguing my mind. *If this is a preview of what's to come in the big leagues, then I am wasting my time.* I wanted desperately to fit in, to make this work, but I had reached my threshold. I wanted no part of the unending mental abuse. I was done. Ready to give up on my dream. To live the rest of my life without ever touching a bat again. I reached for the phone. The receiver seemed to weigh 20 pounds.

"Aubrey?" My mom's voice on the other end seemed happy to hear from me at first, but she sensed something was wrong, and with a little prompting, I let it all spill out. I bellyached to her about everything. I told her how I hated the culture down in Miami, how the guys were so coldhearted, how I just didn't fit in, blah, blah, blah. I'm sure at that moment she wished she had a husband around to offer priceless nuggets of manly wisdom to a son so desperate to hear them.

I kept waiting for words of understanding from her, something to the effect of, "It's okay, son. At least you tried. Come on home." But they never came. I continued to ramble on with excuses. Deep down, however, I knew the truth. I was scared to be alone for the first time in my life and had absolutely no idea how to handle it. No one had ever taught me how to stick up for myself or fight back. I needed to face my fears.

I have recently begun speaking to groups about my life, and God's hand in it. My testimony, if you will. My first real speech was to well over 200 men at my local church men's retreat. And you know what? I was deathly afraid that I didn't have what it takes. The voice in my head drove me nuts. *Who are you to speak about God, Aubrey? After all the rotten things you've done in your life, you are going to stand in front of all these men and speak of God's love for you? Stop it, Aubrey. You're just embarrassing yourself. You will never amount to anything!*

Standing at home plate in front of 40,000 people seems less daunting than speaking in front of a few hundred men to me. When I suited up for the game throughout my career, I felt like I had armor on, and my whole team stood like an army behind me, ready to do battle. I felt safe with a bat in my hands. Speaking from the heart, alone, with none of that support behind me still terrifies me.

A question on *Family Feud* a few years ago was, "What is your greatest fear?" 100 people were surveyed, and the number one answer was public speaking. Number two? Death. I can see why. I certainly thought I was going to die the first time I spoke in public, and never wanted to set foot in front of an audience again. In fact, it took a lot of courage and perseverance to overcome my fear and finally start to get better at public speaking. I had to step right up to my fear and face it head on. It's not something that comes naturally for many of us, but facing your own fear is something I highly encourage you to do.

Everyone has fears. Everyone hears those voices telling them they're not good enough. I heard a great quote by ex-Army Ranger turned fitness model and motivational speaker, the late Greg Plitt. He said, "When we face our fears we become the person we want to be. Energy is never lost, it's transferred. So when we face our fear head on, we beat it. And what replaces it? Confidence."

Before I could overcome my fears and finally grow into the man I feel God wants me to be, I had to first empty myself of all my pride and sense of control. I had to have a childlike faith and trust that when I stepped out onto a stage God would give me the words to say. This was very difficult for me. I always believed that handing control over meant I was weak. But I was wrong. I have now discovered that surrendering like that not only allows me to overcome my fears, but gives me a euphoric feeling that is far better and longer lasting than the high from any drug. I don't believe I can overcome fear in my own strength. Sure, I can handle almost anything for a season or two, but making changes that last a lifetime calls for something, someone, far stronger than me.

This is how I grew. But it did not come naturally, and let me just say I truly wish I understood this concept back in Miami all those years ago!

I was done whining to my mom. The phone went dead silent as I waited for her response...something life-changing. She cleared her throat, and with the kindest, but sternest voice she could muster said something I'll never forget. "Aubrey, if you don't tough this out, you'll never forgive yourself. You'll always wonder 'what if?'"

She may as well have been talking to the wall at that point because I had already thrown in the towel. I was homesick. "I'm done mom. I'm coming home." She could tell I was done talking about it, but insisted she fly out to help me pack and drive back. She booked a one-way ticket to Miami for that coming weekend.

I know why so many people don't live their dreams. I heard a great quote the other day, "If you want to achieve your dream, you have to get comfortable being uncomfortable." It was so easy for me to just quit when it got hard in Miami, and I felt an immediate sense of relief afterward. Like the weight of the world had been lifted off my shoulders. But that feeling is a trap. It felt good right then knowing I dodged the bullet and did not have to face my fear, but now I know that I was just setting myself up for even more pain, regret, and guilt in the future.

I wasn't willing to be uncomfortable. Waiting for me back in Texas was a safe life, joining many of my old high school buddies in the oil fields, making just enough to pay the bills and put food on the table for my future wife and kids. A family I knew I wouldn't be able to lead, because I wasn't a real man. I was a quitter.

My head exploded with the pros and cons of my decision. *Is quitting really what I want? Do I want to go back to a life without passion in Texas?* But baseball was causing me pain, and I wanted to run as far from it as possible. 1600 miles back home sounded like the perfect distance.

As I was replaying my escape plan in my head, I started thinking about what I was going to tell my coaches. *Should I just skip out in the middle of the night?* I knew in my head that my baseball days were done. I'd tried it. I'd given it my best shot. *Time to move on,* I thought. As soon as I got home, I'd tear down that batting cage and live a slow, boring, normal life.

I didn't have a Plan B. I always figured that would distract from Plan A: being a Major League Baseball player. As adults, we are tempted to tell our kids, "You had better have a Plan B for your life." But just because our dreams may not have panned out, doesn't mean theirs won't. My philosophy was to always be "all in," leaving nothing on the table. I chased my Plan A with all of my might. Kids' imaginations are pure. They have not yet had to live in a world of rules, shattered dreams, and disappointments. We must encourage them to dream big and go for it while they still can

I was busy racking my brain, trying to craft a Plan B now, ready to give up on my dream. Then something happened that would alter my destiny forever.

It was Friday night. My mom would be landing the next morning. I had finally worked up the courage to break the news to my roommates. "I'm leaving. Miami just isn't the right fit for me." Kevin's response was the confirmation I needed that I was making the right decision. "Good, we really didn't like you anyway. We need guys here that have balls." I certainly didn't feel like I had a pair, that's for sure. But at this point, I really didn't care what they thought. I was glad that this would be the last day I would ever have to see or speak to them.

Saturday afternoon rolled around. My mom arrived at the apartment at the perfect time. Nobody else was there, thank goodness. My plan was simple. Get packed and get the hell out of there before the guys got home to get ready for the college formal dance later that night.

Packing was moving a little too slowly, and before I knew it, it was five p.m. I heard the apartment door slam shut. "Damn!" My plan was foiled. I had no option now. I uncomfortably introduced Kevin and Ryan to my mom. They shook her hand, looking at me in disgust, disappointed she was there. I felt as low as a cockroach.

We were pushing six o'clock by now. Everything was almost packed and ready to go. One or two more boxes, and we'd be ready to hit the road. I was looking forward to the long drive back home to Texas with my mom. The conversation, the scenery. I have always enjoyed a long road trip.

Pat Burrell's voice was unmistakable as he came waltzing through the front door to pick up Kevin and Ryan for the formal. My mom and I were in my bedroom ready to go, just waiting for them to leave. Having my mom there and knowing I was minutes away from being done with that joint had put me in a better mood. The last thing I needed right then was to see more faces or hear the ridicule as I snuck out with my tail between my legs. My bedroom door was locked. Just another couple of minutes now, and Miami would be a distant memory for me.

Just then, a loud knock on my bedroom door jolted me out of my good mood. My heart started to race. I sat there for a second. *What do these guys want now?* I thought. I flung the door open, ready to face the ridicule that was sure to be on the other side. There stood Pat, completely nude. I could tell by the look on his face he was confused to see an older woman sitting at the edge of my bed. He stood there dripping wet, a six-pack in his left hand,

and an open beer in the other. He didn't even flinch. He looked back at me with a look of disapproval and said, "Hey man, you got any soap?"

I was shocked to say the least. And pretty embarrassed my mom had to see that. I didn't say a word. I just glared at him with as much venom as I could muster and slammed the door in his face. In Texas, you could get shot for doing something like that. Feeling vindicated, I turned to my mom and whined, "See what I have to deal with here, Mom?"

Now my mom is not one for funny one-liners, but her response surprised me. She had this odd look on her face. She just shrugged, laughed, and said, "You know, honey, for a guy that big, you'd think he'd be a bit more endowed!" We both laughed until it hurt.

A wave of realization washed over me. If my own mother could see humor in that, a guy just standing there with his johnson out, then maybe I was being a bit too uptight about this whole thing. Maybe I just needed to take a deep breath and rethink my next steps. That deep belly laugh must have been what I needed. Mom and I sat there and talked, kinda like we used to when I was younger, before I ventured off to Vernon.

The guys went to their formal. We had the place to ourselves. Mom sat there and listened without judgment. I felt like this was truly my decision. That she would support me regardless of what I decided. She helped me look reality in the face and realize that what I had there was an amazing opportunity to pursue my dream.

Months later in the University of Miami locker room, I thanked Pat for that moment. In reality, I now know that there are no coincidences in life. God had to snap me out of it the only way he could reach me at that moment in time. He had to shock me out of my pity party with something pretty dramatic. To this day,

Pat and I always get a good chuckle out of that story. Although he would argue that the hot water in the shower was busted and that is what caused the shrinkage.

As I waved good-bye to my mom at the airport that next day, I also waved bye to the mama's boy version of me. I had made up my mind to man-up. But how? I had never tried being anything but myself, and I knew the real me was an absolute pansy. I knew that if I was going to fit in at Miami, I had to take on a whole new persona. So I created my own alter ego right then and there. My Tyler Durden's name? Huffdaddy.

Something just clicked in me that following Monday at practice. Nothing had changed physically about me, just my mind-set. I decided to stop giving a damn about morals. No more boy scout Aubrey. I was a new man with a different attitude. It was time to have some fun and be a part of the team. That week of practice went a lot smoother for me. Guys were amazed during stretch when I was actually talking trash back. I think I surprised myself. I started to see looks of approval from many of the guys and finally felt like I was going to be okay.

Huffdaddy was invited to one of the famous baseball dorm parties by my best friend to this day, Russell Jacobson.

Huffdaddy walked into that baseball party with Russ that night, and his eyes were opened. Amazed at what he saw. A small three-bedroom dorm room with three tapped Bud Light kegs and a fully loaded bar with any drink you could imagine. It was nine p.m., and a few guys on the team that lived in the dorm had arrived early. They were playing a drinking game called Turtle Master. A memory game challenging you to recite a ballad of tongue twisters without messing up a single syllable. If you did mess up, you had to take a big gulp of beer. Here in its entirety is the sequence players had to memorize and recite. One slip and I'd be chugging.

One fat hen,
Couple duck,
Three brown bear,
Four running hare,
Five fat fickle females sitting sipping scotch,
Six simple Simons sitting on a stump,
Seven Sinbad sailors sailing, sailing the seven seas on a sloop,
Eight egotistical egoists echoing, echoing egotistical ecstasies,
Nine nibbling Nubians nibbling, nibbling on nuts, gnats, and nicotine,
10, I never was a turtle master or a turtle master's friend,
But I'll be a turtle master until the very end.

I was plastered just a few hours later, just as the rest of the partygoers arrived. I'd been drunk before, but this took intoxicated to a whole new level. The next thing I remember was around one a.m. The party was still going strong, and for some unknown reason some of the guys on the baseball team were now completely naked, walking around the party like this was a nudist colony. They coaxed me into stripping down as well. The old me would have said no way, but Hufffdaddy had no fear whatsoever. I stripped down with absolutely no shame.

Now mind you, there were probably about fifty people in and out of this party, and I'd say 70 percent of them were women. Nonetheless, we walked around completely naked with the utmost confidence even though most of us had no reason to be, including myself! I had never felt so free, so alive. All I can think of now is I'm glad there were no smartphones back then. No doubt a lot of us would have been trending on Twitter.

It must have been around three a.m. when I glanced over at a group of people playing cards. A certain player, who wishes to remain nameless, was holding court with a dip in his mouth, playing cards and sitting buck naked on the couch. All of a sudden, I saw everyone around the table jump up, yelling in disgust. Then I saw the reason. He was still sitting as a clear stream of hot urine was shooting out of him onto the coffee table and all over the floor. He didn't even flinch. He just had this stoic expression on his face, as if he'd done this many times before.

Wow! This team truly doesn't give a damn, I thought to myself. *How the hell can this program be so good at baseball when guys are getting this wasted all the time? And more importantly, how can they succeed when they are all this weird?*

From that night on, I truly felt like I was a part of the team. The routine was different for me now. Baseball by day. Party by night. Oh, and we did mix in a class or two every now and then just for good measure.

It's amazing how quickly things changed for me. I started having fun again. Baseball once again became easy the minute Huffdaddy was born. I was cruising through fall baseball practices, hitting better than I ever had before. I was drinking every night, but that only seemed to make me play better.

The Miami Hurricanes were ranked nationally in the top 10 as the spring baseball season approached. And we sure acted like it. I was part of the cockiest, most fun-loving group of guys I've ever been around. The Southern gentleman with the Southern drawl was dead. In his place, my newfound alter ego stood proudly.

As a kid growing up in Texas I always believed God was up there somewhere, and I still did. However, I was living my life and having a good time doing it. *None of us are perfect,* I reasoned, *and once my college career is all over, I'll turn back to the real me and get back to him.* For now, I was the master of my own universe. I would make it all happen on my own.

We destroyed teams on a weekly basis. Not only on the scoreboard but verbally. We talked so much trash, we mentally handicapped other teams. You no doubt have heard about the Miami Hurricanes 1980s football teams that would basically trash-talk their way to countless victories. Well, we were a lot like that. Teams didn't even stand a chance.

That season we made it all the way to the College World Series in Omaha, Nebraska. We had the utmost confidence that we were going to win it all. College baseball isn't quite as glamorous or as big as college football. So the coolest thing for me was getting to play on ESPN as they covered the College World Series. I grew up watching *Baseball Tonight* on ESPN, and now I couldn't help but think some kid out there was watching our games dreaming of becoming a major leaguer, just like I had.

To our disappointment, however, we had an awful series lasting only three games in a two-game elimination tournament. A disappointing way to end one of the best baseball seasons of my life.

That night, Russ and I found ourselves at a local bar playing darts, drinking our sorrows away, trying to push the elimination out of our minds. About an hour in, two of the most attractive women I had seen in all my life walked into the bar. They looked like girls straight out of a country music video. Both had blue eyes, long straight blond hair and were equipped with matching cowgirl hats. They were wearing incredibly tight jeans, with bare midriffs showing off their slightly toned six-pack abs. And, of course, boots. These two were definitely fitting the Nebraska cowgirl profile. Our tongues were on the floor. All eyes in the bar were on these two. They were knockouts and they knew it.

Playing it really cool after our dart game and with miles of liquid courage running through us, Russ and I went over to them, bought them each a drink with our fake IDs, and started chatting it up. The only time I really had any balls to go talk to any woman was when I was buzzed, and on this particular night I was a smooth operator. These girls were young but looked 25. They acted like it too, they were very sophisticated, a lot like Russ and me! I could tell they were taking a liking to us, for some weird reason. I couldn't help but feel like this was the night I was going to finally lose my virginity.

Our alumni group was throwing a huge end-of-season bash at the team hotel outside by the pool, and it was my bright idea to invite the girls to crash it with us. Soon after, Russ and Huffdaddy walked proudly out toward the hotel pool arm in arm with our newfound lady friends. The pool area was full of high-ranking alumni and front office personnel. We didn't spot one single teammate, but that did not deter us. The night belonged to us, and we were about to seize it!

We stepped confidently toward the pool bar, ready to order drinks for the ladies. We were rudely interrupted by one of the nosy front office ladies, Tammy, whose reputation was just that. Nosy. She boldly asked, "What are you guys doing up so late? Who are these women? How old are they?" Before Russ and I could even get a word out in our defense, Tammy very aggressively like a mother hen told the ladies, "Sorry girls, this party is for the Miami Hurricanes baseball program only!" The ladies walked away in disgust. We tried desperately to undo the damage, but it was too late. We watched as they hopped in a cab and disappeared into the night, taking with them the first real chance I had ever had for ending my virginity. I was beyond mad!

We retreated to the pool area to finish our beers and chat about our missed opportunity. I saw Tammy approaching out of the corner of my eye. She was about 10 feet away when I stood up, turned, stared right at her, and with a vicious flash of anger said, "Piss off, Tammy! Don't even think about coming over here to apologize. You've already ruined our night!"

I had barely finished my sentence when I heard a terrifying sound and saw our head coach, Jim Morris, headed straight for us. "Aubrey Huff, get over here!" I shuffled toward him, head held low. The entire party was muted. Anxious to see what would happen. Russ snuck away without detection. Coach Morris grabbed me by the arm and pulled me back inside the hotel, marching me toward the elevator as he let me have it.

"You will not represent the University of Miami like that, Aubrey Huff; you will be disciplined!" The elevator door closed on us. In a smug tone I replied, "Yeah, Jim? I'm one of your best players. Besides the season's over, what are you gonna do about it?" His face turned beet red as he searched for words that never came. He just stared at me the entire way up the elevator. I got out on my floor, fumbled with the room key and finally sank into bed for a sound night's sleep.

The next day on the bus to the airport, Coach Morris called me up to his seat. I sat next to him, no doubt still reeking from the night before. I remembered enough of our little altercation that I figured I was about to get a stern talking-to. To my surprise it was a lot worse than I could imagine. He looked me dead in the eye and said, "Aubrey, your actions last night were beyond embarrassing. You've brought shame to your family and your school. You should be ashamed of yourself. I will not tolerate this kind of behavior at the University of Miami. I have reached out to the powers that be and was told we have a legal right to kick you out of school." I felt like I was going to throw up! He continued, "Instead, I have made a decision to not increase your scholarship for your junior year as punishment for your actions." This would no doubt sting my mom financially.

I went back home to Texas later that week scared to death to face my mom. To my surprise, she actually took it fairly well even though she was disappointed in me. She insisted on me getting a summer job to make up for my stupidity and to help pay for the tuition I had just lost. That one night was definitely not worth it!

I realized then that even though I enjoyed being Huffdaddy, he was a guy that I had a hard time controlling. He seemed to spit in the face of all moral conduct. He was cocky, brash, fearless, and really, really stupid.

I had time to reflect that summer in Texas as I swept floors, scrubbed toilets, and stocked shelves at a local sporting goods store. I am now glad to have had that job, even though I was absolutely miserable there. I quickly learned that there was no way I could ever make it in the real world. A nine-to-five job with a boss who was no older than me telling me what to do for seven bucks an hour? I thought to myself, *How the hell can people live like this their whole life?* No way was I going to let that happen to me. I would rather kill myself than work at a job I had no passion for. I was going make it to the big leagues! Period! But if I was going to make it, I had to bring the partying back in check for sure. I made a vow that summer to quit drinking.

Miami, Junior Year.

My well-intentioned goals were quickly thrown out the window the minute I arrived back on campus for my junior season at Miami. I really didn't like who I was sober. I was such a candy-ass! No confidence and very few social skills. Alcohol was the only thing that made me feel like I had control. I just had no idea what else to do, so Huffdaddy was once again unleashed. The peer pressure was too great.

Baseball Junkie

We were absolutely steamrolling teams from the very
beginning of the season, and spent the entire year in the national
top five. Pat, of course, was our fearless leader. Russ and I were
dubbed the trailer-trash brothers, and our friendship grew even
closer. I finished my junior season as a first team All-American
(the best first baseman in college baseball), hitting a robust .412
with 21 home runs and 95 RBIs, the RBIs a school record that still
stands to this day.

My confidence was at an all-time high. I had even finally found
myself a girlfriend. I met Marissa earlier that season. I remember
it so well because it seemed just like something out of a movie.
I was playing darts with the guys at The Tavern, sipping back
pitchers of Bud Light, when I felt this presence. I turned to
look toward the door, and as if in slow motion, this tall, exotic,
gorgeous brunette walked toward the bar. Our eyes met almost
instantly through the sea of people. She shot me a flirtatious grin.
I tried to pick my chin up off the ground.

She sat at the bar with a friend. I couldn't focus on the dart
game and was glad it was finally over so I could walk over,
introduce myself, and buy them both a beer. I could tell by her
body language she was definitely inviting me to get to know
her better. Marissa was of Cuban descent and an aspiring model
at the time. I could tell she liked to party by the way she was
smoking cigarettes and throwing back the beers; this girl really
knew how to have a good time. I was in trouble!

This was the first real relationship I'd had, and I instantly
fell head over heels. We were no more than a month into our
courtship but I was already thinking about our future together.
Marriage, kids, the whole deal. I was moving fast. Too fast for her
liking. I absolutely smothered her, spending every minute of free
time with her, completely ignoring my teammates in the process.

The season wound down and we found ourselves once again heading to the College World Series. Our last game in Miami was to be played in a regional tournament on our own turf at Mark Light Stadium. We shattered a national regional record that game, hitting 28 home runs. Pat and I had five apiece. I think both Pat and I knew even bigger, better games were in our future, we had no clue just *how* big. We headed to Omaha more than confident this would be our year.

We were heavily favored to win the national championship with all our offensive firepower as the 1998 College World Series began, but in the great game of baseball, anything can happen, and it did. We mustered only two home runs in three games. Pat hit one. I hit the other. Again, we were bounced in just three games, headed home way earlier than we thought we deserved. We were sure this would be the last time we all played together. In fact, for many of the guys on the team, that would be the last time they ever played the game. Back then, the MLB draft was held during the College World Series, not exactly great timing by MLB as players tried to focus on winning a national title. Obviously we were more excited at the prospect of what team would draft us and give us the most money! We all knew Pat would go first round, question was when. I, however, had no clue when I would go.

In our locker room just before our elimination game in Nebraska, Pat found out that he was chosen first overall pick by the Philadelphia Phillies. He instantly became a millionaire. I found out the next day I was drafted in the fifth round by the Tampa Bay Devil Rays. We would both sign, say good-bye to the University of Miami, and hello to the minor leagues.

Now that my professional baseball career looked to be on track, I quickly had to figure out a way to make Marissa and me work. She was only a sophomore, so she still had a few more years in college, but I was determined to figure out a way to make our relationship last.

I don't know what I looked forward to more as I looked to my future. Playing pro ball or not having to go to class ever again! By being drafted, I had taken a huge step toward accomplishing my dream of playing in the big leagues. I knew the odds against me were still massive, but as Dexter Yager once said, "When the dream is big enough, the odds don't matter."

CHAPTER TEN
HORSES*** CITY

"Behind every great man
is a woman rolling her eyes"

—Jim Carrey

I spent eight years with the Tampa Bay Devil Rays organization. I definitely had my ups and downs there, with some of my best seasons statistically on really bad teams. But the Rays were very good to me all those years and helped lay a foundation for my future success. I have fond memories of my coaches and teammates. Baubi, the kids, and I still visit and enjoy the beautiful bay area when we get a chance.

My stats still rank among the best in the club's history to this day, and some would even argue I was one of the best power hitters the Rays *ever* had. But the stats don't tell the whole story.

I showed up in 1998, fresh out of college, and was immediately assigned to the Rays Class A ball affiliate, then the Charleston RiverDogs in North Carolina. I officially signed my contract and began my minor league journey just after the All-Star break that year. My transition to using a wooden bat was smooth sailing, and I had zero trouble with A ball pitching. I finished that year confident I would be moving up to Double-A in Orlando the next season.

My relationship with Marissa was getting rocky that offseason. I could tell she was beginning to drift, and in some ways so was I. I was still head over heels, but halfway through my first minors season, I began to realize there were way more fish in the sea.

As I reported for duty in the spring, I learned I would indeed be starting the season at Double-A Orlando. Playing my first long 148-game season in Double-A would be a challenge for sure, but I was ready.

Marissa continued to drift...all the way to Amsterdam. She had called me to let me know she was going to study abroad, and even though I knew then that that move would mark the beginning of the end for us, for some reason I wasn't ready to let go. I convinced her to give our long distance relationship a shot. It was a nice idea, but it didn't last long.

It was around four p.m. and I was busy packing my bag for Orlando just before spring camp broke. I was missing Marissa and wanted to hear her voice. It was 10 p.m. in Amsterdam, so I figured she should be home and awake. I was shocked to hear a male voice pick up on the first ring. "Hello," a deep male voice with a strong European accent answered. "Is...umm...Marissa home?" I stammered. The guy on the line hung up on me.

I was caught off guard, but called back right away. Again, the phone picked up on the first ring, except this time it was Marissa who answered, "Hello?" My response was pretty measured considering just how furious I was. "Who the hell was the guy that just answered?"

Her reply just rubbed salt in the wound for me, "What guy?" She had barely finished speaking when I heard the same male voice, with the same accent yell in the background, "I'm her new man." He laughed diabolically and trailed off.

I heard Marissa shush him, but it was too late. It felt like a knife had just been plunged into my chest between the second and third rib on the left side, and whoever had stabbed me was now cruelly twisting the blade with all his might. I was crushed. I wanted to punch something! I vowed right then to never ever let any woman hurt me again, focusing only on getting to the big leagues and enjoying the off-field fruits of the baseball lifestyle.

I don't want to sit here and bore you with the details and stats of the next two years of my minor league journey through Orlando and Durham. That would just be cruel. Just know that I partied hard and played hard, in that order. I was breezing through the stops on the way to the big leagues with little to no effort. *If the majors are going to be as easy as the minors, I am going to be one wealthy man!* After a successful double A campaign in Orlando, I was invited to my first big league camp the following spring.

Comparing minor and major league spring training is like comparing a Volkswagen bug with a fully loaded Rolls Royce. I was so happy to be invited to train with the big boys, but did not know what to expect. Any expectations I *did* have were blown away the minute I set foot in my first big league clubhouse. Peanut butter and jelly sandwiches were replaced with all-you-can-eat buffets. My locker wasn't made of chicken wire. Brand new spikes, pants, socks, hats, and bats were already set up in my locker waiting for me, along with my very first big league jersey. And I didn't have to pay for any of it!

I was getting dressed to take the field, still taking in the scene when the traveling secretary walked up to me and handed me an envelope. It was full of crisp hundred-dollar bills—$700 worth.

I looked up at him, confused, and said, "Hey bud, I think you got the wrong guy. This doesn't belong to me."

He gave me the most condescending little laugh as if I were a six-year-old kid. "Aubrey, that is your meal money for the week. You'll be getting 700 more next week. Welcome to the show, kid!"

I sat there staring at the fat wad of cash sitting in my hands in disbelief. I had just made more in one week than I had ever made in a whole month in the minor leagues! I was excited to be there and worked hard to make a lasting impression. I definitely held my own that spring and felt like the big league staff noticed. But I knew I hadn't made the squad. I would be starting the season in Triple-A Durham.

Spring was officially over, and as I stuffed my clothes into an oversized duffel bag, I felt an overwhelming sense that it wouldn't be long before I got called up to the big club. After all, the Tampa Bay Devil Rays were a perennial last-place team. This was a golden opportunity for a young prospect like me to come up and show what I could do. My dream was so close, I could taste it.

Durham, North Carolina, is definitely one of the most beautiful cities I visited in my minor league travels. I absolutely loved everything about it. From the weather and the scenery, to the gorgeous, historic baseball field. But the best part about Durham was nearby Chapel Hill, party place for University of North Carolina students.

Minor league baseball is a very confusing time. I found myself at an age where most men are starting out on their respective careers, getting their first job so they could work hard the rest of their lives just to make ends meet. Here they were struggling to get a foothold in life, while I stood just within striking distance of instant millions.

I'll never forget the day *the* call finally came. It was August 1st, 2000. I hadn't let my cell phone out of my sight since leaving spring training. I knew I had nothing more to prove in Triple-A, especially when I was hitting .316 with 20 home runs, and 76 RBIs. It was a hot day with a summer humidity that hung around like only those who call North Carolina home can relate to. It was an off day around noon, and my mentor, teammate, and good friend Ozzie Timmons knocked on my apartment door, trying to convince me to make a beer run. It did not take a lot of arm-twisting. The plan was to spend the day by the pool at our apartment complex, relaxing, trying not to think about baseball or anything in particular. Ozzie offered to drive. We had made it halfway to our favorite liquor store, about a three-mile run from our apartment, when the phone rang in my pocket. It was my agent. I smiled and took a nervous breath.

"Hey man, what's up?" I said, trying to act all casual. He was trying to surprise me, but his tone left little to the imagination. He blurted out excitedly, "Huffy, I've got great news!" I knew immediately. He didn't even need to finish the sentence.

Ozzie knew too. He beamed at me. "Congrats, kid! Let's toast a few of these beers before you go."

I was excited and scared to death at the same time. Those celebratory Bud Lights never tasted sweeter knowing my minor league journey was over. Or so I thought.

I boarded the plane the next morning ready for my debut in Tampa. I found out I'd be starting that night at third base against the Cleveland Indians, pretty ironic since my favorite baseball movie of all time was *Major League*, a comedy about that same baseball team that I had watched over a hundred times. Dave Burba would be making the start for the Indians. Burba was a very accomplished right-handed veteran pitcher. But he wasn't the overpowering type. *I might have a fighter's chance.* Even so, fear and doubt flooded my mind.

I had seen countless guys get called up to the big leagues only to be back a week later. Would I be one of them? I was an all-star in Triple-A that season, but being an all-star in the minors means jack squat to anyone in the big leagues. Part of me wanted to just ask the pilot to point the plane at Texas so I could go home and forget the whole deal. But the words my mom had spoken to me when I wanted to bail on Miami years earlier rang in my ears. I knew this was something I had dreamed about my whole life, and I would never forgive myself if I didn't stick it out. Still, I had never been more nervous in all my life.

I landed in Tampa about one p.m. drenched in sweat. I headed straight to Tropicana Field, the armpit of Major League Baseball stadiums. A huge, dirty white dome sits over Tropicana Field, shielding the hardest, most fake-looking artificial grass from the blazing Florida sun. The atmosphere and fan base rivals that of most high school baseball games. It has been consistently ranked as one of the worst stadiums in Major League Baseball. But to me, it might as well have been heaven!

I rolled my bag into the clubhouse, nervous, not sure what to expect, only to be met by clubhouse manager Chris Westmoreland. He looked at my bag. He looked at me. Then he took the bag from me as if to say, "Son, you have no business carrying that heavy thing!" He hauled it straight to my locker and promptly began unpacking it, hanging everything up neatly. This was certainly new in my experience. To be honest, I felt pretty uncomfortable standing and watching someone else doing my dirty work.

I didn't stand there for very long, however, because I was summoned to manager Larry Rothschild's office. He greeted me and went over my role for the rest of the season. The meeting was quick. But I still walked out of his office a nervous wreck.

I walked around the clubhouse and shook hands with several of the guys on the team that I had met just months prior in big league camp. I exchanged pleasantries with Gerald Williams, Greg Vaughn, Steve Trachsel, John Flaherty, Vinny Castilla, Tony Graffanino, Ozzie Guillen, Tanyon Sturtze, and Randy Winn that day. I also couldn't wait to see one of my favorite veterans of all time by far, Fred McGriff aka "The Crime Dog." Fred was a kindhearted man with a serious streak of comedic sarcasm to him. His Eddie Murphy–style laugh was infectious. He called me over to his locker.

"Hey kid, you okay? Looks like you're gonna puke." He no doubt knew exactly what was going on in my head.

"Yeah man, I'm a little nervous, that's all."

He chuckled, "Well, I wouldn't worry about it too much, Huffy. If you suck, you'll just go back to Triple-A."

With this, he walked off, laughing in his trademark chuckle. *If he's trying to comfort me, he's doing a terrible job,* I thought. But he did have a point. *Worst case scenario, if I do, in fact, suck, I won't die. I'll just go back to Triple-A.* My nerves calmed down, if only for a few minutes.

Batting practice was about to start. My first as a Major League Baseball player. As I strolled out to that field for the first time to stretch, I felt a sense of peace and calm. *My dream has finally come true,* I thought to myself. I had to fight with everything I had to not cry tears of joy. The anxiety of that morning was replaced by a sense of accomplishment, happiness, thankfulness, and gratitude.

That first batting practice felt like a true breath of fresh air. You see, in the major leagues you are expected to be professional, on time, and to do what you have to do to get yourself ready to play. You create your own program, so to speak. You hit extra if you wanted to. You lifted weights if you felt like it. You are treated like a man.

Gone were the days of being treated like a peon in the minors. Of always having to show four inches of sock between the bottom of your pants and your shoes. Of being clean shaven, with facial hair that under no circumstances goes past the cut of your lips. The minors are all about control. You have to be at a certain place at a certain time, or else. You have no say in anything. It was the organization's way or the highway. Moving from that environment to the professional atmosphere in Tampa felt like I was a kid at a private boarding school finally let off his leash. As we began to stretch down the right field line at Tropicana Field, only half the team was in attendance. The stretching basically consisted of the guys sitting around, chatting it up. I was amazed.

The most defiant guy on that team by far was Jose Canseco. Jose was a real treat to watch day in and day out. He would dress as if he was stuck in the '80s and was absolutely jacked. By his own admission later, he had been using steroids for years. He had an ego unlike anything I had ever witnessed in the game. He simply strolled everywhere he went as if in no big hurry. He wasn't a jerk to me, but I can honestly say I don't remember having one conversation with him the entire time I was his teammate. I was basically nonexistent in his eyes. But he sure was fun to watch. His daily routine walking into the clubhouse was lackadaisical at best. He would head to his locker, trade his wardrobe of skintight clothing, clothing that showed off all his muscles in all their glory, for more comfortable team attire. He would then head to the training room, and sit back on the training room table while the trainers attended to his every need.

We finished stretching and it was finally time for batting practice. Jose finally decided to make his appearance, strolling out of the dugout with a little more pep in his step. I could tell this was his favorite part of the day. He hit in the first group and I was hitting in the third, so I was able to watch this power display with utmost amazement. I never knew a human being could hit a ball that far. From the first swing he took in batting practice to the last, he had one thing on his mind, and that was to see how far he could hit a baseball. It was and still is to this day the most impressive performance in batting practice I've ever seen.

As the game inched closer and closer, my nerves almost got the better of me. I was at the peak of my anxiety. I would be hitting seventh in the lineup that night and playing third base.

Six fifty-nine p.m. *Just one more minute till we take the field.* I paced nervously back and forth in the dugout. Fred McGriff came up and put his arm around me, "Remember, kid, don't suck."

Our starting pitcher Bryan Rekar led us out onto the field. I followed, my legs so wobbly I almost tripped over the dugout stairs. I stood at the hot corner playing bunt defense with Kenny Lofton leading off for the Indians. My legs were still shaking so bad I could barely get into defensive position. All I remember thinking was, *Please don't hit it to me. Please don't hit it to me!*

Thankfully, my prayers were answered. I made it past the first two defensive innings without a play. Now it was my turn to hit.

I strode to the plate for my first major league at bat leading off the top of the third inning. "Batting seventh, number 37, third baseman Aubrey Huff." I wondered silently, *How the hell am I gonna be able to swing the bat?* I was so paralyzed. I stepped into the left-handed batter's box and unconfidently looked in Dave Burba's general direction. I had no intention of looking him in the eyes to size him up. I felt unworthy, like an unconfident freshman in high school trying out for the varsity baseball team.

I knew beyond a shadow of a doubt that he was going to challenge me with a fastball, but I had no intention of swinging. I wanted to see what a major league pitch looked like before I swung at one. As he began his windup, I couldn't slow my heart rate down. Breathing became a chore. His fastball couldn't have been any more down the middle at 89 miles per hour. In the back of my mind, I knew I could have hammered that pitch like I had countless times in my minor league journeys.

Even so, I was still petrified as I gathered myself for the second pitch, trying desperately to breathe easy and slow down the endless assault in my head. The next pitch I guessed would be another fastball, so I inched back into the batter's box. Indeed it was a fastball on the inside corner. I had every intention of swinging, but as the pitch came, my legs were still shaking so bad and my heart racing so fast that I couldn't get my brain to tell my body to swing. Strike two.

I felt weak and overmatched. I stepped out of the batter's box to gather myself, but the negative thoughts were relentless. *I'll never make it. I'm not good enough. Will they send me down?* Fear was paralyzing me. I felt like the entire stadium was whispering, "Why didn't he swing at those two fastballs right down the middle? What's he waiting for?"

With all that was going on in my head, I needed to find a way to calm down. Then I remembered who was sitting 15 rows up behind our home dugout down the first base side. I turned to look up into the stands to catch a glimpse of my mom, grandma, and grandpa. I remembered all the sacrifices they had made to help get me to this point. The proud look on their faces gave me the courage I needed to step back into the box and take a rip. Dave threw his best changeup, and I gave my best swing, grounding out to first base. Even though I grounded out, as I was headed for the dugout, I thought, *Well, at least I swung.* Moral victory, I reasoned.

Even today, I'm amazed when I see a guy making his major league debut getting a hit in his first at bat. I always wonder how they did it. Weren't their legs shaking? Are they just mentally stronger than I was? More confident?

I once again grounded out to first base on my second at bat off Dave Burba. Only this time, to my embarrassment, his 87-miles-per-hour fastball on the inside corner absolutely shattered my bat leaving it in dozens of pieces in front of home plate. 0-for-2. *I'm going to be sent down for sure,* I thought.

I went up to the training room to get my new bat some grip tape the next inning. Jose Canseco sat on the training room table talking on his cell phone. A television was playing the game in the background. Jose was the designated hitter that night, the one guy on the team who hits but doesn't play defense. In my opinion, DH is the best job on the planet! While I was taping up my bat and watching the game on the television, I noticed that Jose was hitting third that inning. I looked back toward him and pointed toward the TV. "You're up."

He looked up at the TV and ever so calmly said to whomever he was speaking to, "Hey, hold on a second, okay? Don't hang up, I'll be right back." He put his phone down on the training room table and walked out, in no particular hurry. I finished taping my bat and hurried behind him to watch what was about to unfold. He arrived in the dugout just in time for his at bat. He grabbed his bat, walked up to the plate with no warmup swings, and proceeded to hit the first pitch he saw for a screaming line drive off the left center field fence for a double! I was amazed! Here I was having a complete heart attack every time I was up to bat, yet he made it look like a walk in the park, quite literally. I always wondered if he went right back to his phone conversation in the training room. I'm sure he did.

It was the bottom of the seventh inning. I walked toward the plate with Canseco on third, and one out. I would be facing a new pitcher in Steve Karsay, a hard-throwing right-hander out of the bullpen. I knew the situation. All I needed to do was to hit a fly ball deep enough to the outfield so I could get Jose in from third with a sacrifice fly. I had worked the count to 2-2. Karsay delivered a fastball on the outside corner. I lifted the baseball deep to the left field warning track, plenty deep to score Jose and to give me my first-ever big league RBI.

I felt like the weight of the world had been lifted off my shoulders. I confidently strutted into the dugout to an array of high fives from my big league teammates. And for the first time that day, I was able to smile.

I was so happy when the ballgame was over even though we lost 5-3. Now I felt I could finally catch my breath and take in the entire day. My dream had become a reality. I could now call myself a major leaguer!

I finished the remainder of that season hitting a respectable .287 with four homers and 14 RBIs in 129 plate appearances.

But 2001 was a different story. I struggled mightily that year, spending my season on a shuttle up and down from Durham to Tampa. I ended the year hitting just .248 with only eight home runs in 111 games. I seriously doubted whether I had what it took to stick in the bigs.

I felt the 2002 season was a make-or-break year for me. Unfortunately, it started with a break. I began the season once again in Durham, and during a batting practice was struck by a baseball in the left temple right next to my eye, shattering my orbital socket. After hours of surgery, two screws, some fine Swiss titanium, and loads of painkillers, I emerged almost as good as new. Only to spend a month on the disabled list.

I wrote earlier that the doctor told me then that if my orbital fracture had been just a millimeter longer, my eyeball would have dropped out, quite possibly making me lose sight in my left eye.

I returned to the Tampa Bay Devil Rays lineup in late May an entirely different player. It was almost like the doctor had given me a bionic eye. I delivered a .313/.364/.520 line with 25 doubles, 23 homers, and 59 RBIs in 494 plate appearances. My swing was back, and I led the Devil Rays in home runs even though I played in just 113 games.

Things were on the up and up on the field and off. That offseason, I met the woman of my dreams.

It was 11 p.m. December 7th, 2002, on a cooler Saturday night in Tampa. I was in my Superman pajamas lounging on my couch watching TV. I was about to fall asleep when I got a call from Pat. I knew he wanted me to meet him out somewhere, but I really didn't want to go anywhere. I fought the urge to answer for a moment, but finally gave in. I'm forever thankful I picked up.

"Damn, Pat. What the hell you want this late?" I asked.

I could hear loud music in the background as he screamed across the line, "Hey man, you have to get to The Coliseum. Gia knows this waitress who is dying to meet you. Trust me when I say you won't be disappointed." Gia was Pat's girlfriend. "I'll be there in 20 minutes," I said, hanging up the phone with a newfound energy.

I found Pat and Gia sitting at a VIP table full of bottles and mixers. "Okay, where is this woman?" He pointed at someone through the sea of people. As if from a movie scene, the lights shone down perfectly on this absolute knockout blond-haired, green-eyed beauty. The sea of people seemed to magically part just for her as she glided toward our table with a tray of shots. I moved my gaze from her hypnotic eyes to her toned, tight body and lean, strong legs. I had never in all my life seen such an unbelievably gorgeous woman!

My heart began to race faster and faster. I tried desperately to come up with something clever to say. She sat the shot tray down and sat down right next to Gia. Gia then casually introduced me to Baubi. I reached out my hand ever so nervously to shake hers. I felt intimidated by her beauty.

"What are you drinking?" she asked.

I needed booze quickly if I was going to have any kind of game with this lovely woman. I answered quickly, "Tequila shots. Make it two. With two Bud Lights. And why don't you open up a tab for yourself tonight, sweetheart, your drinks are on me." Cheesy, I know.

She walked away to get the drink orders and returned shortly after, this time sitting right next to me, fully waiting on me to start some kind of conversation. I was desperate.

"So, do you like baseball? I play for the Devil Rays, you know. Would you like to come watch me play one day?"

She looked at me dead in the eye with a disgusted look, "Umm no. I hate baseball." She took her shot, got up, and walked away.

Pat, of course, witnessed the whole thing and was dying laughing, "Well you blew that one, didn't ya, cowboy?" But I wasn't going down without a fight.

Throughout the course of the night I was finally able to convince Baubi I wasn't a tremendous douchebag. You're probably seeing a trend in this book by now. Despite myself, and by some great miracle, I got Baubi's telephone number.

Now I have to say at this point in my life I was pretty success-ful with the ladies and didn't have to work real hard to get dates. But Baubi, on the other hand, made me work overtime to earn her adoration. It took almost a month of begging and pleading to finally get her to say yes to a first date.

Baubi was different than any other girl I had ever met. Yes, she was obviously gorgeous, but better yet, she was fun, exciting, adventurous, smart, and had a touch of danger to her. And we both loved to party. We began to get serious in a hurry. She was obviously the woman for me. As a matter of fact, she proved to be my lucky charm. In baseball there is an old saying, "If she has hits in her, keep her." Well, Baubi certainly did.

That next season in 2003, I became an offensive force not only on the Rays but in the entire major leagues, with a slash line of .311/.367/.555. My 47 doubles pegged me third overall in the American League, and my 198 hits earned me a respectable fifth. My .311 batting average and 34 homers both ranked ninth. I also drove in 107, setting the franchise record for RBIs. For my efforts that year, I finished 24th in Most Valuable Player Award voting. This, despite playing for a last-place team. My efforts that season were rewarded with a brand-spanking-new, three-year, $15-million deal.

I knew exactly what I was going to do first with all that money. It was time to keep my promise and pay my mom back! Two weeks later on a gorgeous sunny Saturday in St. Petersburg, Florida, I picked my mom up at her rental home at nine in the morning. She had moved to Tampa a few years before to be closer to me, and now she had absolutely no idea what I was up to. She sat excitedly in my car, just like I had all those years back when she had taken me to my first Rangers game. Our first stop was the Ford dealership. I glanced over to see her face as I pulled into the lot. She had a smile on from ear to ear. I walked up to the first salesman I saw and proudly told him, "Get this young lady whatever she wants."

My mom is such a Texan! Of course she would pick a Ford Explorer Sports Trac, a spunky little maroon truck that fit her perfectly. As we were in the sales office signing the papers, an uncontrollable wave of emotion hit my mother. She began to cry uncontrollably with tears of joy. *She hasn't seen anything yet!* I thought to myself.

She sat in her brand new truck. "I have one more surprise for you." I told her to follow me down the road.

We drove for about 10 minutes toward the water in Largo, a small suburb of St. Petersburg. I pulled into the driveway of a quaint two-story 2,100-square-foot home just walking distance from the ocean. My mom was so overwhelmed, she almost ran into me in her Sports Trac. The real estate agent was waiting for us, and as she handed the keys to my mom, she warmly said, "Welcome home, Mrs. Huff." That was more than my mom could bear. Her tears ran like rivers.

Seeing her tears made me realize just how far we had come since I made that promise as a nine year-old. The realization that my dream had actually come true made my eyes begin to water. It was one of those surreal moments that felt like a dream.

Not much changed for the rest of my Rays years from 2004 to 2006. We continued to suck, finishing at the bottom of the American League East standings. And I was still putting up solid offensive numbers.

I had purchased a small townhouse in the Saint Petersburg area in 2002. It was the first house I ever owned, and it still holds a special place in my heart. Baubi and I had fallen head over heels for each other, and she moved in.

My life was going great. Almost *too* good. Baubi and I were a passionate couple. We fought hard and loved hard. My mom was taken care of. My baseball career was rocketing skyward. I had made millions before my 30th birthday. But one thing was missing: I was ready to start winning.

On July 12th, 2006, I was shocked to learn I was traded to the Houston Astros. The Astros were in the thick of a playoff race when I arrived, and I held my own during my time there hitting .250 with 56 hits, 10 doubles, 13 home runs, and 38 RBIs. However, it wasn't enough. We finished a game and a half behind the St. Louis Cardinals for the National League Central title. I filed for free agency immediately after the season.

January 2007 was a very happy time for me. I signed a three-year, $20-million contract with the Baltimore Orioles.

And that same month, on the 27th, I married the love of my life, Baubi.

I did not exactly earn my $20 million salary that 2007 season, batting just .280 with 154 hits, 34 doubles, 15 home runs, and 72 RBIs. I also managed to upset a lot of Baltimore fans that following offseason.

Baubi and I had gotten in a pretty big argument, and I felt the need to take the day away from her. My destination? A gentlemen's club off Kennedy Boulevard in Tampa called The Doll House. At this point in my life I was certainly buying in on all this world had to offer. I was young, successful, good looking (in my opinion), and had loads of money. To put it simply, I loved me some me! I was polishing off my ninth Bud Light around one p.m. when I got a call from a good friend and radio DJ Matt Loyd. Matt asked me if I wanted to come on to his show and rap about life. The station was right around the corner from where I was, so I agreed. I should have known better. His show was called *Bubba the Love Sponge*. It was a Howard Stern–type of syndication. Obviously in the state I was in, not a good call to go.

I sat down some 20 minutes later with Matt and Bubba feeling pretty good after drinking more than a few Bud Lights. We rapped about life and what it was like to be a major league baseball player. Now keep in mind this show is a shock-jock type of environment.

Bubba asked me, "So Aubrey, do you like Baltimore?" I slurred, "What a horse**** city." I was really just playing into the shock-jock deal and left the studio thinking nothing of it.

The next morning my phone woke me up at seven a.m. "Huffy, what the hell did you do?" my agent yelled through the earpiece.

Confused, I asked, "What are you talking about, man?"

"Go online to *The Baltimore Sun* and call me back after you see the front of the sports page."

I immediately hopped out of bed and stumbled into my office computer. I pulled up *The Baltimore Sun* website, and there it was, first story of the day in big bold lettering, Huff calls Baltimore horse****!

I had to make all kinds of apologies. The Orioles organization was going as far as threatening to take away my deal due to a morals clause in my contract. But they never pursued it. The best apology any player can give isn't words. It's performance. And perform I did.

I posted one of my best statistical campaigns batting .304 with 182 hits in 154 games. That record tied my teammate Nick Markakis for 10th in the league. I also hit 48 doubles, 33 home runs, and 108 RBIs. If you just look at the statistics, you could be forgiven for thinking I am just bragging here. But as any player will tell you, there is a lot of heartache, pain, and disappointment that lives between each of those numbers. The failures and struggles make your achievements and recognition as a player taste even sweeter. I finished sixteenth in American League MVP voting and was named Most Valuable Oriole by Baltimore sportswriters that year. This was also the year I won the Silver Slugger Award as a DH and the Edgar Martínez Outstanding Designated Hitter Award.

Baltimore introduced me to newfound recognition for my hard work. I achieved new highs in my career there. It also introduced me to my first taste of a high of a different kind. Adderall.

So by now, I have told you about my childhood and high school experience. I have brought you up to speed with my career spanning the University of Miami days, all the way through the Baltimore Orioles years. You know about my short stint with the Detroit Tigers right before I signed with the Giants. But I guess I am best known for my two World Series wins. This is where we will pick the story back up.

CHAPTER ELEVEN
PAPI'S RALLY

*"There's got to be
more than this."*

—Tom Brady (after winning his 3rd Super Bowl ring).

October 7, 2010.

Back in San Francisco, I settled into that calm before the storm. A chance to let my mind and body heal from the grind of 162 games. Right before the chaos, that if we were lucky, would last for an entire month.

The sound of my alarm that morning brought a fresh wave of nervous excitement with it. Pent-up frustration that had steadily built up steam for almost a decade of losing was finally over. The time had come.

I had no idea what to expect. I could barely get anything down for breakfast. I did, however, make sure I washed down 20 milligrams of Adderall with a cup of coffee. My morning vitamins to take the edge off.

One pill was barely enough to settle my nerves these days, but as I waved at the gatekeeper and pulled into the players' parking lot, the anxiety, fear, and nervousness I had felt an hour earlier were now a distant memory. In their place were confidence, excitement, and a feeling of invincibility.

I parked my car in the players' lot underneath the stands of the left field bleachers. I wanted to take a different path today instead of my usual track through the concourse toward the clubhouse. I chose to take the scenic route, walking through the green gate down the left field line. I wanted to experience firsthand what the stadium looked like dressed and ready for playoff action before I ingested the remainder of my 60-milligram dose. Red, white, and blue half-circle banners hung off every railing in the place. *Someone spent some time hanging those*, I thought. It felt like the Fourth of July. Like something big was about to go down.

The right field archway would typically sport the scores of all 30 teams in the league. Now, I noticed only eight teams listed. *Just eight teams.* The full weight of the importance of it all began to sink in. I stood there for a minute taking in the scene with a cool bay breeze blowing in my face, enjoying the peaceful silence in full gratitude of the opportunity before me. I walked down the dugout stairs, through the dugout, and headed for the clubhouse, knowing it was about to be a madhouse.

The San Francisco Bay Area alone boasts a population of over 7,000,000. It was surprising to me that such a storied franchise hadn't won a World Series for the city. Playing as the New York Giants, the team had won 14 pennants and five World Series championships behind managers such as John McGraw and Bill Terry. Legendary players like Christy Mathewson, Carl Hubbell, Mel Ott, Bobby Thomson, and Willie Mays had helped build the Giants into the stuff of legends. But that had all ended with the move to the West Coast in 1958. Yes, 52 years was a long time to wait for even the most dedicated of fans, and I was thrilled at the idea of being a part of the team that had a real chance of ending that drought. A chance to become a legend. This was going to be epic for San Francisco. And for me! To say fans were excited would be a gross understatement. Tickets were being scalped at over $1,000 each just for the opening game.

I now understood that special playoff "electricity" fellow pro players speak of. That magic you feel only if you have experienced the madness firsthand.

There was a huge difference in the atmosphere that morning. I felt it the minute I walked onto the field for batting practice. Playoff banners hung everywhere. Media crawled over almost every inch of the stadium. There was a new vibe in the air. Something I had never felt before.

The National League Division Series determines which two teams will advance to the National League Championship through a best-of-five series, and we had drawn the Atlanta Braves for game one and two at home. Two-time Cy Young Award winner Tim Lincecum got the ball. Here we go. Nothing like ripping the lid off a brand new playoff series! Definitely a new sensation for me.

After what seemed like an eternity, it was almost game time. Each player was introduced individually as our teams lined up down the first and third base lines respectively. With the announcement of each player's name came a huge roar of the crowd. Call me crazy, but the roar following my name seemed the loudest. I fought back my emotions. Every hair on my body stood on end. It was electrifying.

The National Anthem raised the excitement to almost unbearable levels. I simply couldn't wait to take the field. I tried to stand still. To listen. To pay due respect to our national anthem. But I couldn't stop rocking back and forth, shifting my weight from my left foot to my right, and back again. I was on drugs designed to control ADHD. Now I was acting like I *had* ADHD! I wasn't the only one. I looked over at the Braves on the first base line and noticed they were all doing the same thing. Every player on that field was amped up to do battle, dripping with sweat, even though the game-time temperature was 61 degrees.

The grind of the past 162 games faded. 60 milligrams in my system. Primed. Amped. Ready. I felt just like Superman, hunched down ready for lift off. I don't think I could even blink. I was locked in.

Finally, after watching a B-52 bomber fly low over the stadium, feeling the stadium shake from its power, it was time to play ball!

Tim Lincecum was locked in the entire game. He completely dominated, striking out 14. A complete game shutout. We won 1-0, the only run coming on an RBI single to left by Cody Ross. We had just picked up Cody on a waiver claim a month earlier, and he was already earning his keep. In fact, in my opinion, this waiver claim would prove to be the best waiver claim perhaps in the history of baseball. I'm not sure what was fueling Cody, but he was simply the hottest hitter on planet Earth during our playoff run. His passion and power helped us finish the Braves off in four games. And he was just getting warmed up.

Now that we had the division series behind us, next in our way were the defending National League champs, the Philadelphia Phillies. We shouldn't have stood a chance in this best-of-seven series. They were better in every way on paper. Every so-called baseball expert had them beating us in five or six games; we were no doubt the underdogs. The Phillies could absolutely mash on offense, something our team had struggled with all year long. However, we hadn't worked this hard and come this far to simply roll over. We knew they had to face our all-star pitching staff. And we all knew that good pitching trumps good hitting any day of the week. Every guy on our team that year will tell you that it sure did not feel like we were the underdogs in the locker room. We were confident and ready.

The first game of the series was in Philadelphia. Once again Lincecum would face off against one of the best pitchers in baseball: Roy "Doc" Halladay. It was an exciting game all the way down to the wire, but we pulled it off with a 4-3 victory, again led by our waiver pickup sensation, Cody Ross. Cody hit two big solo home runs off Doc Halladay, turning the game in our favor. The newspaper headlines the next day pointed out that Cody Ross spelled backward spells "Sorry Doc!" We took that as an omen.

The Phillies weren't going to make it easy for us. They evened it up the next night just in time to move the action back to San Francisco for the next three games.

We won the first two games in exciting fashion. We were now up three games to one, with one more game to be played at AT&T Park before heading back to Philadelphia to finish the series. Obviously we didn't want to make the five-and-a-half-hour flight back into hostile territory. This was a game we desperately wanted to win. We wanted our celebration to be in front of the greatest fans in sports.

Game five started off well enough in front of a raucous crowd of 43,713 fully expecting to party that night. We had a 1-0 lead going into the top of the third. With runners on second and third, and one out, the Phillies' Shane Victorino stepped to the plate. When you're on defense, you have to go over every scenario in your head before it happens, and I knew exactly what I was going to do if it was hit to me. I was playing medium depth at first. If a ball was hit hard to me, I would check to see if the runner from third was headed home, then I would try to throw him out at the plate. If it was hit slowly, I would just take the sure out at first. Sure enough, Shane hit me a hard grounder that I took my eye off for the slightest of seconds to check to see what the runner at third was going to do. That split second cost us. The ball completely missed my mitt and ricocheted off my knee into shallow right center field, scoring two runs. To make matters worse, Victorino was able to get into scoring position at second base due to my error. The next hitter, Placido Polanco, singled to left center, scoring Victorino. Phillies were now up 3-1.

We ended up losing that game 4-2, and I felt like I wanted to puke. That error cost us the game. I thought of all the fans in the stands and the countless people at the local bars let down by me. I thought of the almost six-hour plane flight we had to take the very next day because of me. I had just added another day, perhaps two, of extra stress for my teammates.

I spent the entire flight to Philadelphia the next day head down, barely speaking to anyone. I felt so ashamed that I had let the team down. My mind was quickly flooding with thoughts that maybe the Phillies would win the next two games, stealing the series from us. I thought for sure if that were to happen, the media, fans, and my teammates would look back at my blunder as a turning point in the series.

Game six couldn't have arrived fast enough. I felt like if we didn't win this game, we would surely be done. We had to win.

It was a pressure-packed game. One of the tensest I had ever experienced. You could feel the momentum shifting in the Phillies' favor. The Philadelphia crowd was even more rambunctious than ever. It was the kind of game where you just knew a big home run was going to win it. And fortunately for us, it did. Game tied 2-2 top of the eighth inning, two outs. Juan Uribe stepped up to the plate and hit a Ryan Madson fastball into the first row of the right field stands for a solo homer. 3-2.

Now, if you have been living under a rock your whole life you could be forgiven for not knowing that the city of Philadelphia and its fans take great pride in being absolutely obnoxious. They boo anyone and everyone, especially their own players. They are a miserable breed of fan, no doubt. They have even thrown snowballs at Santa Claus. I'm sure there are many decent people in the city, but I have only met a select few.

Fans in Philadelphia would wait outside our hotel, getting ready to follow and heckle us unmercifully any time we stepped out for a lungful of fresh air or to go anywhere. They obviously didn't have a life, and got pleasure out of making derogatory comments about our families. I will never forget this one particular scumbag. He looked like he was in his late 20s, obviously still living in his mom's basement, and by the looks of him, eating everything he could get his hands on. Not sure if his mom's house had running water either, because he looked like he hadn't showered in days. He was smelly, looked disheveled, and was wearing clothes that were a size too small and hadn't seen the inside of a washing machine in a month. This guy was about as charming as a cockroach, and about as smart too. I am sure he would have crapped his pants if I confronted him, but the slimy prick must have felt pretty brave hiding behind his camera phone, knowing I would stand to lose millions if I engaged him.

He followed me around for a good 15 minutes, filming me as I made my way from the hotel to a restaurant where I was meeting Pat Burrell for lunch. He spent the entire time verbally assaulting me in his obnoxious incoherent Philly accent, baiting me, desperately waiting for me to react so he could catch me on video attacking him.

I treated him like the cockroach he was and just walked on, not even acknowledging him. His frustration grew as I continued to ignore him. He inched closer, yelling, "Aubrey, your dad was shot because he was a p***y like you!" I must admit, in that moment I could fully understand how someone could commit murder. My blood ran hot. I knew that one clean punch would have smashed his nose in and sent him running back home to his mommy. But I knew once I started, I wouldn't stop until he was dead. Thankfully, somehow, I was able to gather myself as I walked through the restaurant door, leaving him behind.

I believe there is a special spot reserved in hell for people like that. Come to think of it, he's probably still living with his mom. Or perhaps he's dropped dead of a heart attack. By the looks of him, he wasn't too far off. Needless to say, I took great delight in the conclusion of that game.

It was the bottom of the ninth with two outs. A runner at second. Brian Wilson, our closer, was up against Philadelphia's dangerous power-hitting first baseman, Ryan Howard.

Closers have a different mentality. They have to have this fearless, insane quality about them. They come at you with some of the nastiest pitches in baseball, holding nothing back. They amp up their persona on and off the mound, almost like a professional wrestler getting into an act designed to get inside their opponent's mind. At six foot two with a huge, jet-black beard and not an ounce of fat on his body, Brian was all that and more. He looked intimidating on the mound, standing wide-eyed with a piercing stare, eyeing the scene like a hawk. Fully locked in. No one worked harder than he did in the clubhouse. He was a great teammate with a huge persona that fed the monster he created. Brian was an animal in the gym and meticulous about what he ate. He wanted to be feared.

So it had come down to this. A one-on-one battle between Brian Wilson and Ryan Howard. There could only be one victor here, and we were all just spectators along with the fans in the stands. As the excitement built to a fever pitch, the stadium vibrated, seemingly louder than usual, if that was even possible. Brian wound up, and Howard watched strike three sail by. The roar of the crowd was immediately silenced. All you could hear was crickets for a few seconds, followed by our celebratory screams as the whole team piled up around the pitcher's mound.

I had waited my whole career for this. The ultimate pinnacle of baseball—the World Series!

As National League champions with 14 competitors behind us on a scrap heap, it was now time to turn our attention to the American League champions, the Texas Rangers, the very team I grew up rooting for. I would be playing in the same stadium I had spent so much time in as a kid, collecting autographs, studying my heroes. But before our trip to Texas, we had to play two games in San Francisco.

Life certainly does come full circle. I knew playing the Rangers was going to be a very emotional experience for me. I had to hold it together. We had business to attend to. A World Series to win.

I stood in the lineup waiting for the announcer's introduction. That playoff opener now seemed like years ago, and I wasn't near as nervous this game. I was quickly getting used to the stress of the postseason.

The Texas Rangers would be pitching one of the greatest pitchers ever to pitch in the postseason, Cliff Lee. Even opening at home, we were underdogs that first game, but we loved having something to prove, and all the pressure was on the Rangers. We came out on fire offensively, knocking out Cliff Lee in just four-and-two-thirds innings. And we didn't let up. We continued with our assault on their bullpen, winning that game convincingly.

Game two was a laugher. AT&T Park was rocking. We won 9-0 behind the strong right arm of our bulldog on the mound, Matt Cain. Our work here was done. Now we were ready to step on the Rangers' throats as we moved the Series to my childhood stomping grounds, Arlington.

Being back in Texas to play against the team I grew up rooting for felt surreal. I paced around my hotel room like a caged animal, game three now mere hours away. My phone and email blew up with messages from people who I hadn't talked to in years looking for tickets to the big game. I distinctly remember many of those same people telling me that I was wasting my time all the way from little league through high school, saying, "You'll never make it." And to stop wasting hours practicing in my batting cage. Needless to say, there were not a lot of ticket requests granted for that game.

Oddly enough, I was not nervous stepping out onto the field. In fact, it felt like déjà vu...like I had done this a thousand times. Again, the announcer started in with introductions. I felt like I was in a dream that I never wanted to wake up from. My childhood memories in that stadium flashed before me. My grandparents and their love for the Rangers. Knowing that if it weren't for them, there was no way I would be standing there right then. I knew they were watching from somewhere above, but I desperately wished they were there in person.

Baubi, Jayce, and Jagger sat with the Texas-side of our family in the stands. My mom, sister, niece, and in-laws, not to mention all of my old friends and coaches, were all there waiting for the action to begin. It took everything I had not to break down in tears.

The announcer's voice rang out, "Batting third, first baseman, Aubrey Huff." I snapped out of it. Game time.

I don't want to bore you with the details of our game three loss. The Rangers' win got them right back into this series. The next night would be pivotal. We knew we had to go up 3-1. We didn't want them gaining momentum, feeling like they had gotten back into the Series. Game four for us was a must-win.

We had everything on the line. And we turned to our baby-faced, rookie man-child, Madison Bumgarner, to shut down the Rangers' high-powered offense. You no doubt know how Madison has dominated the game in recent years. The man is an absolute badass on the mound and in life. But keep in mind, this was his first World Series game. He was just 20 years old and in hostile territory.

We knew the kid could pitch, but weren't quite sure he had the mental game down yet, or the focus needed to keep it together under the immense pressure he was sure to face that day. The kid didn't even break a sweat as he steamrolled through the Rangers' offensive machine. He shut them down in a hitter-friendly ballpark, making it all look so effortless. Here he was, a small-town, hardworking country boy from North Carolina playing with the big boys. And he showed absolutely no fear whatsoever.

I loved hitting in American League ballparks. I especially loved to DH in them. Many players don't like to DH, saying they don't feel "locked" into the game. I, however, loved to be the designated hitter. The way I saw it, if I were the DH, I could only be a hero, not a goat. If I struck out with the game on the line, well hey, hitting a baseball is the hardest thing to do in sports! A critical error at first, however, would be replayed and remembered forever.

I would be facing Texas Rangers' starting pitcher Tommy Hunter that day. It was the top of the third inning, and as I strode to the on-deck circle, I couldn't help but remember hitting countless balls in my batting cage all those years ago as a young man just miles up the road, visualizing myself hitting a home run in the World Series at the ballpark in Arlington. It was something my mind had seen clearly thousands of times with every single pitch coming at me from the machine. A majestic homer right down the right field line. I was more than mentally prepared for this moment.

Time passes and you forget about all those dreams and visions you had as a kid, but not today. Not for me. Those dreams and sensations came flooding back to me all at once. I was overwhelmed with emotion, realizing that I had an opportunity to make that dream a reality.

Andres Torres, our spirited spark plug at the top of the lineup, had just led off the inning with a double. A strikeout by Freddy Sanchez was my cue to stroll up to the plate. The score was 0-0. The next minute played out in slow motion.

Tommy started his windup with his first pitch to me. Everything was moving pretty normally, but as soon as the ball left his hand, it was as if it was floating toward the inside part of the strike zone. It literally looked as big as a watermelon as it inched toward me. I was ready to pounce, and swung the bat with textbook speed and accuracy at just the right time. The ball met the bat, but I never even felt it. All I heard was that magical sound of wood to baseball and the groan of the crowd. As I watched the trajectory of the ball down the right field line, I knew it was gone. I stood to admire it just long enough to not show anybody up and to make sure it stayed fair. The ball landed 50 rows back in right field. It was about as far as I could possibly hit a baseball. Exactly like in my vision.

I took off, rounded first and headed for second base in a leisurely jog. I felt like I was walking on air, just like when I hit my first big league home run almost a decade before, on August 10th,

2000 off Jason Ryan of the Minnesota Twins. I took in the silence of the crowd. My right foot hit second base and I looked up to the second deck, right above the third base dugout. As I rounded for third, emotions overcame me. That was the exact spot I remember eating hot dogs on all-you-can-eat Thursday nights with my mom and sis, rooting for my Rangers. I could smell the hot dogs, the fresh-cut grass. I could feel me. Looking back down onto the field...at me!

The next thing I remember I was back in the dugout celebrating with my teammates. I must have mentally blacked out because I don't even remember touching third base or shaking the third base coach's hand. Time stood still. My mind was in such a state of ecstasy and emotion that I don't think I could have even spoken if I tried. You have no doubt heard the corny saying, "If you can dream it, you can achieve it." Well, it was in that moment that I became a serious believer.

As I sat replaying the home run later, I realized something. As a kid, visualizing myself hitting that exact home run a thousand times, I never really stopped to think about the jersey I was wearing. I had always just assumed I hit that homer as a Ranger. Good thing for the city of San Francisco that I didn't!

We won that game 4-0 and were now enjoying a commanding World Series lead over the Rangers. Three games to one. Just one more win, and we would be champions.

November 1st, 2010, will be a day I'll never forget. As a kid, when you play a sport and you want to become a professional, you never think of the money, the fame, the material things that come with it. All you think about is winning that championship. That ring that has eluded many hall of famers from all sports. It truly is a rare thing to reach the pinnacle of your sport, but it is even rarer to win a championship ring. So it was on this day that we would be going up against Cliff Lee once again, with a chance to bring the first World Series trophy home to San Francisco.

It was a pitchers' duel with Tim Lincecum once again dominating in a 0-0 game. Leading off the top of the seventh inning, Juan Uribe and Cody Ross got back-to-back singles off Cliff Lee, putting runners on first and second, with nobody out. Up to this point of my 10-year major league career, I had never been asked, nor had I ever attempted, to sacrifice bunt. Now I was being called to do so off one of the best left-handed pitchers of our time. Since I'm a left-handed hitter, it was a simple call for Bruce Bochy to make. I didn't really even need to check the signs from our third base coach, Tim Flannery. I understood the situation. I had to advance Juan and Cody. I knew the only option was to bunt.

Cliff threw his fastball up and in, a perfect pitch to bunt, and I bunted it perfectly between Lee and the first baseman. If I ever had a chance to make it to first off a bunt, this would be it. I ran like hell thinking, *Maybe I can make it.* But Cliff Lee is a tremendous athlete, and he leapt into action, making a great play to just barely get me out at first. But I had done my job, moving up the runners to second and third with one out.

I had set up my good friend and old University of Miami teammate Pat Burrell with the opportunity to drive in the winning runs that would seal the deal for the championship.

I could almost see the headlines now: "Pat the Bat's big stick wins Series for Giants."

There was no doubt in my mind that Pat was going to come through. It was just too perfect of a script. However, it wasn't in the cards. Pat battled in an epic at bat that ended with him striking out on a 3-2 pitch. Now, Cliff Lee was just one out away from getting the Rangers out of serious trouble.

But Lee would have to face veteran shortstop Edgar Renteria next. Edgar's RBI single off Charles Nagy in the 11th inning of game seven back in 1997 won the first-ever World Series for the Marlins. He had earned himself a World Series hero badge with the Florida Marlins back then, and now he was looking to do the same thing for the Giants a full 13 years later.

The count was 2-0. Cliff Lee had a base open at first to work with. I leaned anxiously over the dugout railing watching what was about to transpire, biting my nails and wondering if he would even challenge Edgar with a fastball in the zone.

Lee decided he would. A decision he would immediately regret. As the pitch sailed in, a fastball up in the zone, Edgar pounced on it. He hit it solidly into the left center field gap, and it looked like at least a two-run double. Even better, however, it kept going and cleared the fence. Three-run home run! The entire dugout went ballistic! And the stadium, absolutely silent. We knew right then and there. This series was over.

The Rangers were on the ropes, and now it was time for our all-star closer, Brian Wilson—"B-Weezy"—to finish them off.

He took the mound for the bottom of the ninth. 3-1. Brian was always the type of closer who could make it scary, but we all knew he would come through for us. He always did. I manned first, trying to get a grasp of the roller-coaster ride that had gotten us to this moment.

I eyed Nelson Cruz as he took a leisurely stroll toward the plate with two outs. He was the Rangers' last hope, but the look on his face gave nothing away. I almost felt bad for the guy at that moment. That's a lot of pressure to place on one man's shoulders. I was praying Brian would make this quick and painless for him, and us! *We don't need any drama,* I thought. *Just get him out. Get it over with so I can finally breathe and celebrate.*

Wilson did not disappoint. He struck out Cruz swinging.

And just like that, we became the 2010 World Series champions!

I charged toward the mound, threw my first base mitt toward our dugout and joined the absolute mayhem at the pitcher's mound. I looked for the one guy on the team I couldn't wait to hug: Pat. We had known each other since college, and now here we were 12 years later celebrating a World Series together. As I was walking around the infield celebrating with the sea of media, coaches, and teammates, I couldn't help but think of all that had transpired in my life to make this moment happen. If only my dad were here to see this. His son. A World Series champ!

I always got a kick out of watching players getting interviewed after winning championships at Super Bowls and what-have-you. There would always be that one guy who lost it. Crying like a baby. I always thought to myself, *Why the hell you crying? You just won it all!* Well, I was about to become one of those guys.

At this point I think the mix of beers and champagne must have started to kick the Adderall back into gear. I was having an absolute blast celebrating with my teammates. As the media closed in around me at my locker, I heard a familiar voice from years past.

It was Tampa Bay Rays beat writer Marc Topkin, a man I respected not only for his writing but for his professionalism. I had spent hours chatting with Marc over the years. He knew me well.

His question to me was, "Aubrey, how does it feel right now as you look back on your life, the tragic death of your father, your mom supporting your dream with the batting cage, the years of losing, and the heartache in Tampa? What does this World Series victory mean to you?"

I could barely get any words out. I starting crying like a baby. It wasn't all the losing in Tampa that made me lose it. It was the thought of my mother and my grandparents. The endless sacrifices they had all made to get me to get to this point. But the biggest thing I started to realize as celebrations died down and the media started to leave, was that I had been so distant from Baubi and my children for months. As a matter of fact I never went outside the clubhouse to the concourse to escort my family in. Most of my teammates' wives and children were running around in the clubhouse celebrating. Not mine. They never even crossed my mind. This was my moment and nobody else mattered. I had completely consumed myself with baseball and myself. I very rarely thought about how my behavior was affecting them. A tremendous feeling of guilt came over me as we headed back to the airport that night.

I dealt with the guilt the only way I knew how. I drank it away on the plane ride back to the West Coast. I was surrounded with an endless sea of happiness on that flight. Yet I felt miserable and alone.

I lay in bed next to my wife the next morning. A newly crowned World Series champ. Hungover. Drained. Sad. Empty and unfulfilled. I turned to Baubi, wiping the sleep out of my eyes, and mumbled, "Hmmm. Now what?"

CHAPTER TWELVE

THE BROTHER I NEVER HAD

*"Things come apart so easily
when they have been held together
with lies."*

—Dorothy Allison

We waved good-bye to our furnished rental home for the past six months, and flew back to Tampa as a family for the 2010 off-season. I remember being surprised by just how much stuff we needed for such a tiny, little, newborn baby, and how much harder it seemed to mobilize the troops now that there were four of us.

As a newly crowned World Series champion, I was expecting to feel amazing, but the feeling from the day after the big win lingered on. I walked around most days with a very dull, unsatisfying feeling. I was still using Adderall, but I had backed off from the 60, sometimes 100 milligrams I was taking during the World Series run. I was a couple of weeks into my offseason, and already I was bored and antsy. The melancholia was driving me crazy. *Why can't I be happy?*

Thinking back now, I am amazed I didn't drop dead of a heart attack by taking that much of the stuff during the playoffs. I knew my body needed a break. I could feel it. But I wasn't about to quit cold turkey. Every now and then I tried skipping it, but on those days, I found myself suffering through a hopeless, miserable, draining, depressing existence. All I would want to do was sleep the day away with nobody bothering me. I knew I was hooked, but frankly didn't care, and would have been fine taking Adderall the rest of my life.

Jayce was now two years old. You would think I would have plenty on my plate, especially with a newborn added to the mix. But I was bored out of my mind. My relationship with Baubi was basically nonexistent. I was cold, distant, non-communicative, unhelpful, and mean. I would fly off the handle at the slightest provocation, often losing it if she asked me to do anything or ask for help with the kids in any way. I was always edgy and couldn't stand still. I constantly needed to be doing something. I had no idea how to relax.

I dealt with the wired feeling by hitting my familiar offseason stomping grounds, the Hard Rock Casino in Tampa five times a week. Sometimes I would win; sometimes I would lose. But I didn't go there to win. The casino was the only place that offered happiness and excitement for me in my reckless state.

There is no doubt in my mind now, that if Baubi and I didn't have kids together, she would have already divorced me. But in my mind, there was no way she was ever going to leave me. *After all, I'm a rich, handsome World Series champion. She'd have to be an idiot to leave me,* I thought. I was a catch, pure and simple.

God knows how to mix things up, and he was about to make life really interesting.

My sister Angela, or "Angie" as I affectionately call her, is three years younger than me. We don't speak that often. I love her to death, like I'm sure any big brother loves his baby sister, but she and I have always struggled to find things in common. Even as kids, we hung out with completely different groups of people. I am driven and social. She is the exact opposite.

I wish I had a better relationship with Angie, but growing up without a dad wreaks havoc on kids, especially a young girl. A dad helps build a girl's confidence, and she was robbed of that. She was three years old when my dad died; I was six. I dealt with my demons through alcohol and Adderall, tools that helped me move away from the gravitational pull of the weight of growing up without a dad, and that made me keep my distance from my family. It hurt less that way. But it also built a wall between my sister and me.

I was a little surprised when she called me out of the blue early one morning. She didn't sound herself, and I have to say my mind raced as I tried to figure out what terrible tragedy had just transpired.

"Aubrey, you sitting down?" I put down my cup of coffee and gave her my full attention. Apparently she had some "big" news for me and didn't know how to break it to me. She told me that mom had received a Facebook message from a woman named Jodi who lived in New York. As my sister read the message, I must say, I found it really hard to believe.

"Hello Fonda,

My name is Jodi, and I am Chris Dickerson's girlfriend. Chris is 36 years old. It took some time to find you on Facebook, but I have some information that could potentially be huge. We live together in New York. And I know this might sound strange, but recently Chris and I were watching the World Series between the Giants and Rangers, and when your son Aubrey Huff was up to bat, the announcers on the television were talking about how when Aubrey was a young man, his father Aubrey Huff Jr. was shot in Abilene, Texas when he was only six years old. When we heard the announcer say that, Chris, and I were in disbelief. You see Chris had a father named Aubrey who he never knew, and he also died, being shot in Abilene, Texas.

And as we went online to read more of Aubrey's story, more and more parallels were the same as Chris'. Not only that but when I put their faces up next to each other, they could be twins! I know this must be rather shocking to you. But I think we need to get these two on the phone together to chat, as I think they are half-brothers. I wanted to reach out to Aubrey, but I'm sure as busy as he is after winning the World Series, he would just think we are someone just wanting something out of him.

This is absolutely not the case. We want nothing from him, only to talk to see if possibly they are family. Thanks for hearing me out, and please let me know if Aubrey would like to talk to Chris. Here is a photo of Chris to show you how alike they really look.

Thanks, Jodi"

My first reaction obviously was disbelief. You see all kinds of things as a pro athlete, and the paranoia that develops in your mind after a while makes you distrust everyone outside your little bubble. I was sure this was a con, someone trying to get money or something out of me. But my doubt faded the minute I saw the photo of this Chris guy. My heart stopped for a second, and a chill washed over my entire body. I felt like I was looking at a picture of me!

I had to know for sure. "Angie, I'll do a DNA test only if he sets it up and pays for it. If he's our brother, we have to know!"

Chris agreed, and two weeks later the results arrived. I felt like I was about to step on stage at *The Jerry Springer Show* as I opened the envelope. I sat there nervous to open it for a minute, feeling the edges of the envelope, just staring at it. Finally, I tore it open. The result? It was a 99 percent match. We were half-brothers! I felt like all the air had been vacuumed out of my lungs as I sank back in my chair.

I didn't know what to say to Chris, but I knew I had to call him to get all the information I could. Turns out Chris' mom, Melody, had been dating my dad right around the time my mom had met him in Texas. My dad was a Navy man and traveled quite a bit, so the encounter with Chris' mom didn't surprise me in the least. Chris' existence, however, did. I found myself half angry and fully confused about the whole situation. How had nobody known about this? I thought, *Did Dad even know about Chris? And if he did, then how could he have kept this information from my mother? My mom must have known!*

It was just weeks before Christmas and with all that was going on I needed to lean on my wife. We both decided on a much-needed date night. It was amazing that she actually agreed as much as she despised me. But she couldn't help but feel for me with the information I just got hit with.

Our date was a tragedy. All I did was slam beer after beer to try and get numb. *Had my mom lied to me all these years? Did my sister know?* I thought. I took my growing rage out on my poor wife. The night turned into a knock-down, drag-out argument as I switched to attack mode. I was in no mood for anyone's opinions or advice.

It was a long drive home as Baubi and I screamed at each other at the top of our lungs. I couldn't wait to get home and go sleep in the guest room. But my night was just getting started.

My sister Angela had volunteered to babysit the boys while Baubi and I attempted the date night. I walked through the door, steaming mad. My sister has not always been the best at timing, and on this night she proved it.

I had just grabbed another beer when she hit me with a bombshell.

She was surprisingly calm and confident as she sat down next to me and said, "Aubrey, I think it's time you know the truth about mom and dad." *Great! What now?* I thought. She had my full attention as she continued, "I should have told you this earlier, but about two years ago I was rummaging around mom's garage and found a box full of old papers. I came across a divorce document. I confronted mom about it and she finally came clean. She told me that she and dad were in the middle of divorce proceedings when he was shot."

As if I don't have enough going on in my life. The last thing I need is this betrayal! I was livid at not only my mom for keeping the divorce secret from me all these years, but now also my sister. She had known for two years and decided to keep it from me! I violently screamed out in rage at her. "I can't believe you never told me about this! Who do you guys think you are? Get the hell out of my house you freeloader!" She left crying. It felt good to see tears streaming down her face.

It was just before midnight. Now it was my mom's turn to feel my wrath. I dialed her number. Angie must have already warned her I was on the warpath because she picked up on the first ring.

I burst out, "You've got some serious explaining to do Mom, I'm coming over right now!"

"Now"? She replied, somewhat taken aback.

"Yes, right now. I'll be there in 45 minutes."

I pulled into my mom's driveway at one a.m., still fuming, and in absolutely no condition to be operating a vehicle.

My mom had sacrificed a lot raising Angie and me as a single mom on a Winn-Dixie salary. She spent years saving so she could buy me a batting cage, and had supported my every step in my baseball career, always encouraging me to follow my dream. Now I decided to repay her by showing up at her house mad and high as a kite. In my mind, she deserved it!

My mom was not necessarily the most forthcoming person I knew growing up, and that had always bothered me. She would always change the subject any time I would ask her a question about my dad or his side of the family. I felt I never got a straight answer from her. Now that I knew about Chris, it all started to make sense. Or so I thought.

I stood at her front door banging loudly and wildly. She answered with a bewildered look on her face as I blew right past her toward the living room. "Okay, tell me everything!" I demanded.

It took her a few minutes. She sat there, a glass of water clenched between her hands at the kitchen table. She took a deep breath.

She told me she didn't have a clue about Chris until just after the World Series. She had received a Facebook message that caught her attention. Apparently she was getting a lot more friend requests ever since my career had taken off. This message caught her eye because the tone was so nice and polite. It was the same message Angie had forwarded to me. And just like I was, she was skeptical until she saw the photo of Chris.

She was nervous to share the news, but was planning to tell me in person after I had a chance to enjoy my first championship. She swore up and down to me that she had absolutely no clue about Chris' existence before that message, and I believed her.

In fact, she had Angie reach out to my dad's nephew and sister to find out what she could. Both of them apparently couldn't get off the phone fast enough when confronted. They had definitely known about Chris, and apparently, so had my dad. But for reasons I will never know, Aubrey Huff Jr. had decided to keep his son Chris a secret from my mom, Angie and me, taking the information to his grave. I could tell that my mom was genuinely hurt and confused, and was struggling to process it all. She gave me a pained, sorrowful look. Yes, the relationship my father had had with Melody was before my mom and dad had met, but I could tell it still hurt her deeply. Seems like my dad had done a lot to hurt my mom. This was just the tip of the iceberg.

The floodgates opened, and all the questions I had stuffed deep down inside of me all of those years came firing out.

"Mom, why have you never talked about Dad? Why have you barely no pictures of him...no mementoes...nothing of his that you can hand down to me?" I was clearly enraged, confused and lashing out at her with venom I had kept a tight lid on for too long. She started sobbing uncontrollably. It should have broken my heart, but I didn't care! I wanted the truth, and I wanted it now.

She finally composed herself long enough to answer all of my questions.

As we sat across from each other for well over an hour, moonlight streaming in through the kitchen window, each of us too emotional to budge out of our chairs, she recounted the years of turmoil my dad had put her through.

She had grown tired of the lonely nights, wondering when my dad was going to come home. Wondering where he was, what he was doing, who he was with, and just how drunk he was that particular night. She had put up with years of neglect and emotional abuse from a man who preferred to deal with his issues with a twelve-pack of Bud. My dad was lost and had pushed everyone away, putting my mom in a terrible position. As a mother of two young children, she had to make a tough decision for our sake, and although she loved my father deeply, she just couldn't live under the uncertainty anymore. She felt she had no choice but to divorce him. To try to find a way to create a new future for us so that we had a chance at a normal life. Turns out the divorce was why my dad moved an hour away to Abilene, Texas, in the first place.

Tears streamed down my mom's face as she explained how they were right in the middle of the divorce when my father was shot. She was distraught the morning she learned the news that she was now a widow and that her two kids were to grow up without ever knowing their dad. But she had to keep it together. Stay strong for our sake.

Even with the way my dad had acted and treated her, my mom wanted to protect him, to have us remember him as a hero, not the man she couldn't stand anymore. Hearing this gave me a newfound understanding for why my mom kept this from me all these years, but I was still angry at her for thinking I couldn't handle the truth. For me, that was demoralizing. Like I had been betrayed.

I got what I came for on that midnight trip to my mom's house. I had asked her to tell me the whole truth about my dad, and got my wish. As it all sunk in, a heaviness washed over me. A profound sadness at my dad's waste of a life.

It suddenly dawned on me. My dad had obviously made some terrible decisions in his life that not only had cost him his family, but ultimately his life. Now I was on that exact same dark path.

Turns out the old saying held true for me. I was a regular chip off the old block!

As my mom sat there crying, I finally felt some closure. I looked up and saw my mom's face transform, as if a huge burden was finally removed from her shoulders. She no longer had to pretend my dad was a great man.

I got up, ready to leave. It was close to three a.m. "Aubrey, I do have something for you. I'll be right back." She returned a minute later. The only two things my mom had kept were his old bowling ball stuffed in a ball bag, and his old medium-size Navy jacket he had worn in the Navy when he was 19. I immediately threw the jacket on. It was a tight fit. Emotions overwhelmed me as I breathed in a scent that immediately transported me to a time long ago. It must have been his scent from before he was murdered. It flooded my conscience, and the floodgates opened. Tears of sadness, pain, and mercy for my dad washed over me.

I forgave my dad that night. I forgave him for never being there for me and for all the things he had done to the family. After all, I had become the same exact guy. I needed to forgive him, just like I needed to be forgiven.

Now I needed to meet Chris in person.

I invited Chris and Jodi to Tampa for Christmas. In the meantime, my mind spun out of control with all sorts of crazy thoughts those weeks. As the days passed leading up to their visit, I found my confusion growing, still not understanding why my dad had kept Chris's existence a secret. I felt betrayed, and that fueled my addictions even more.

I tried to learn as much as I could about my half-brother before his visit. Chris had made a name for himself in New York as a successful opera singer and is very talented. The more I learned about him, the more I couldn't wait to meet him in person.

What should I do when I meet him for the first time? Shake his hand? Give him a hug?

I paced anxiously at the bottom of the escalator at the baggage claim in the Tampa airport. Finally, I saw him coming down. I knew it was him. There was no mistaking him. He spotted me halfway down the escalator, and we both smiled uncomfortably. Again, I was not really sure what to do, but he walked right up to me and grabbed me, lifting me up in the air, giving me the biggest, sincere, warm hug I had gotten in a long time.

"Nice to meet you little bro," he said excitedly as he continued to hold me in the air. His excitement was evident; he was so happy to have a brother. I, on the other hand, was still very confused and felt really awkward. This was just happening way too fast. I knew he was my half-brother, but I wasn't really sure how I felt about it.

It was a very awkward Christmas Eve for me. And whenever I felt awkward, I would just drink more and use. Instead of hanging out at my house with my family and getting to know my brother personally, I decided to get really high. I even had Chris and Jodi take an Adderall with me. Once the drugs hit us, we were like old pals. We all decided it would be a good idea to head out on the town to party. Our destination? The Doll House, a gentlemen's club in Tampa.

My wife was repulsed, and I don't blame her. As I look back at it now, I realize how incredibly sad and disgusting that decision was. At this time of my life, God was not even a blip on my radar. Instead of celebrating the birth of Jesus with my wife and gorgeous boys, I would be tipping dancers 20 bucks at a strip club. I was a confused and lost soul, desperately trying to fill that void in my heart and numb all the confusion in my head.

The next morning, three of us woke up with hangovers. Christmas Day. We sat in the living room around the tree opening presents, my wife not even looking or talking to me. Who could blame her? I flew Chris to my home to get to know him, and we had spent the entire time drinking and partying. Not really a great way to get to know someone. All I knew for sure after those few days was that we were definitely brothers. He liked to party like I did. Like Dad did. Chris was a huge Crown Royal fan, and ironically enough, when I was in the mood for whiskey, that was my favorite as well. I really did enjoy spending time with Chris. Once the initial awkwardness of the first day or so left, it really was like I had known him my whole life. I wish I would have.

2010 was a whirlwind year for me, and as it came to a close, it felt bittersweet. What an emotional roller coaster! I needed a time-out. To get away. I had to escape to Vegas for a few days. Clear my head.

I turned to Russ. It took some convincing, after our previous trip to Vegas, but thankfully, after he heard about my dad and half-brother, he agreed to make the short plane trip out from Scottsdale. My friend Ralph, the card counter from California, agreed to join us as well.

As soon as I landed and turned my phone on, I saw I had a message from my agent. I had an opportunity to make a quick 25 grand the next day at a card show signing in San Jose, California. Was I interested? *Let's see,* I thought. The flight from Vegas to San Jose was literally an hour. *One-hour flight there, one hour signing autographs, one hour back. 25 grand minus 6K for a private jet leaving 19K to throw down for blackjack.* The math worked!

Russ beat me to the Bellagio, but Ralph wouldn't be arriving until the next evening. Russ and I made a night of it before I had to fly out to San Jose the next morning. I invited him to go with me, but he decided to stay back. So that morning I threw down my pill, grabbed a coffee, and headed to the airport dressed to the nines, looking like the same rock star who had walked into Brian Sabean's office in Scottsdale a year earlier. I don't remember a time in my life when I felt more confident. But it wasn't a natural confidence, it was a confidence shrouded in insecurity. The drugs seemed to bring out the man in me.

The limo ride from the Hayward Executive Airport to the San Jose convention center took no time. The sign hanging from the building said "Sponsored by Hooters." That should have been the first red flag. Mistake number one: I didn't turn around and head back to Vegas.

As I walked to my signing table, I noticed dozens of Hooters waitresses fully equipped in the patented Hooters outfits walking around greeting patrons. I sat down and went about my business, signing what must have been 500 cards in 60 minutes. My work here was done. I shook hands with the guy running the table and headed to the front of the building. I spotted four Hooters girls on a smoke break, and did what every man asking for trouble would...I headed over to join them. Mistake number two.

If I had a time machine and could go back in time to change just one thing about my life, this would be one of those idiotic moments I would like to erase.

We got to talking. They knew who I was as we talked about baseball and the playoffs. Huffdaddy, the egotistical monster inside me that fed off the least bit of attention or adoration, was in heaven. The girls saw my limo pull up and asked me where I was headed that day. Without hesitation I said, "Vegas. You guys want to come? I have a jet leaving in two hours." I didn't even have to twist their arms. They jumped at the chance and promised me they would be at the airport just in time for takeoff.

What the hell was I thinking? Now I'm one to own up to my mistakes, and I have made my share of screw-ups, and this one has to top the list. I should have lost my family and friends over the decisions I made during that 24-hour period. I regret those decisions deeply to this very day.

Please understand that I'm not trying to glorify my behavior. As a matter of fact, this is very hard for me to put down on paper. Whenever I think about it, I have an overwhelming feeling of shame, guilt, and disgust at myself. There isn't a day that goes by where I wished I never let the Adderall and booze take over my life. But it happened. And I can't blame the drugs or booze because it was my decision to let them in. I made my own bed.

As the jet touched down in Vegas, I texted Russ and Ralph: "I have a surprise for you guys." Russ had agreed to meet me down at the Bellagio main bar while we waited for Ralph. And so in I strolled down the Bellagio lobby, a newly crowned World Series champ, dressed in full midlife-crisis gear, two Hooters girls on each arm. It seemed like all eyes in the casino were on us. Incognito, I was not! Russ's disgusted look of disapproval told me exactly how he felt.

Like me, Russ was a married man with a beautiful wife and two kids at home. And he was having absolutely none of this! Like the good friend he is, he pulled me aside, looked me square in the eyes, and told me, "Dude. I love you. But you are blowing it!" He told me I was a completely different man than he ever remembered, and that he just couldn't be friends with me anymore if I was to continue down this self-destructive road.

I was surprised by his tone of voice and seriousness. I honestly had no bad intentions with the women. I was just at a point in my life where I thought that this would make a cool story someday. I thought I was cool, and having Hooters women walking around with me would make me look even cooler. Obviously I was not thinking very rationally. I was a complete scumbag. I was so lost, it makes me cringe just thinking about it.

How was I any different than my old man before me?

I made plans to meet up with the ladies later at the Hard Rock. They took off to go check out the town. Russ decided to get on the next flight home back to Scottsdale. He wanted no part of what I had going on. We hugged. And he headed up to his room to pack. I should have done the same. Mistake number three: I didn't.

I sat at the bar nursing a drink, waiting for Ralph to arrive. When he did, we didn't waste any time. We exchanged pleasantries, then immediately ditched his bag, and headed straight to the Hard Rock to begin counting at blackjack. By the time the girls arrived, we were up a good 30 grand and feeling great. I'm not going to go into details about the rest of the night, you can use your imagination. Let's just say I'm not proud of the decisions I made that particular evening.

As my Vegas trip ended, I headed home heavy with shame, and ridden with guilt and regret. And just like my dad before me, I justified it all in my mind, making up an elaborate lie for when I got home to my wife. Little did I know that I would be walking straight into an ambush.

I knew the minute I stepped through the front door that Baubi was not herself. She stood there with a glass of water in her hand. I'm sure it would have been a martini had she not been nursing Jagger. She seemed on edge as she followed me into the kitchen, asking me very calmly how the trip was. "Great!" I responded. I gave her the highlights, bragging about the 30 grand Ralph and I had won, and how well the card signing in San Jose had gone.

Not a minute later, she hit me with it. "I'm going to give you a chance to tell me the truth, Aubrey. Tell me the truth and I might forgive you." My heart began to race. *What did she know? What was she talking about?* I could never tell her the truth. It would break her heart and would surely be the last straw for her. So I said, "Baby, we just gambled and drank the entire time."

She gave me one more chance, and stupid me...I just repeated my previous answer. She put the glass of water down, took a deep breath, looked me in the eyes with an intense stare and said, "Tell me about the Hooters girls." My jaw dropped to the floor, utterly speechless, with a look like I had just been caught with my hand in the cookie jar.

Staring into her sad, tired eyes I could literally see her heart break as she reached for her water and splashed it in my face. Her face turned red with a mixture of anger and pain as she screamed at me, "Aubrey, you're a pathetic excuse for a man! I'm leaving you and I'm keeping the kids! I want you out of my house now. We're through!"

CHAPTER THIRTEEN

WINTER IN SCOTTSDALE

"Sometimes God lets you hit rock bottom so that you will discover that He is the rock at the bottom."

—Dr. Tony Evans

I stood there furious, shoving clothes into a zip-up bag. *How did Baubi find out about the Hooters girls?* I focused the blame on anyone but myself, burning with anger at whomever had ratted on me. I was consumed with rage and a determination to flush the rat out. I didn't even stop to consider how I had betrayed my wife and kids.

I checked into a studio hotel room a few miles down the road, and had barely walked through the door when I got a call from Ralph. "Be careful with your wife, Aubrey. My wife just got done wearing me out about the trip." He said his wife had called him while he was out on the Vegas Strip with a couple of the Hooters girls. Apparently he didn't hear the phone ring in his pocket, and it answered without his knowledge. According to his story, his wife listened to every single thing that was said for a full 20 minutes. Ralph said his wife was threatening to call Baubi.

"Too late dumbass," I said. "She must have already done that, because Baubi kicked me out." I hung up. Paranoid thoughts dancing in my head. Something about his story didn't add up.

I mulled it over for a few minutes and decided that it must have been Ralph himself that had rolled over and ratted me out. *What kind of friend does that?* I felt so betrayed. *What was I thinking? What kind of an idiot trusts a card counter? A professional cheat!* That would be the last time I would ever speak to Ralph.

Two weeks had gone by, and I can't say I was enjoying my stay at the hotel. It did, however, give me time to calm down and start thinking about my juvenile actions. I would alternate between blaming Ralph for throwing me under the bus and feeling true remorse for the pain I had caused my wife. *I have to kick the Adderall,* I thought.

Baubi was kind enough to let me still see Jayce and Jagger when I wanted to. She didn't have to do that, and I really appreciated it because I missed Baubi and the kids terribly. I begged and pleaded with her to take me back, and each time I got the exact answer I deserved, a big "Go to hell." But one time, the answer was a different one.

I drove over to the house one night to hang with the kids, and after I tucked them in, I made my way to the living room, and sank into the leather recliner. She sat on the couch across the coffee table. With absolute sincerity in my heart I laid my soul bare. I told her how much thinking I had been doing. And that I had now realized that it was the drugs that were doing this to me. I promised her I could change. That I *would* change.

I could tell she was torn. I knew she didn't care to have me back in her life, but for the sake of the boys, she thought about what I was saying for a bit. I must say Baubi is a far more considerate and forgiving person than I could ever be. I knew I didn't deserve a 20th chance, and I was not sure that I would have given her the chance were our roles reversed. She must have seen something good deep down in me, even when I couldn't see it. After all I had put her through, she pushed her feelings aside. "The only way I might forgive you, is if you go to rehab," she said. I couldn't believe what I was hearing.

My mind raced as I drove back to the hotel. I was excited to get a whiff of hope. I didn't want to go to rehab, but I knew deep down that this was my only chance to get my family back. Problem was, spring training was starting in less than two months. The clock was ticking.

Baseball was certainly the last thing on my mind that offseason. In just a couple of months, I had gone from being crowned a world champ, to finding out I had a half-brother, to finding out my dad was just as big a wreck as me, to finding out my mom was in the middle of divorcing him when he died, to getting kicked out of the house myself. And now, I was headed for rehab!

I got busy looking for options. The only logical choice seemed to be a rehab place somewhere near Scottsdale, Arizona. In my mind, I'd check into a prison cell for thirty days, check the box, then when I was done, I would immediately head to spring training camp. To join my brothers as we prepared to defend the World Series title.

I looked for a facility that had a gym so I could stay active, but with no luck. The next best option seemed to be a place called Sundance with a shuttle to a local public gym twice a week. But the biggest reason for the decision to attend Sundance was that it had a separate VIP wing for so called "celebrities" like myself.

The previous season had been the best of my career, and in November the Giants had signed me to a brand new, three-year, $30-million deal. This was a nice hike from the original $3-million bargain-basement discount I joined them at just a year before.

On paper, my life was perfect right then. My baseball career was on fire, and I was famous now. But that fame felt fake. Shallow. Like an empty lie. A lie I had been living my entire life. My personal life hung around my neck like an anchor. *Maybe rehab is what I need to kick-start my life again.*

The previous season I was a vocal leader on and off the field for the Giants. Every guy on that team became an instant legend in San Francisco, and I, in particular, was one of the free-spirited veteran leaders and fan favorite. I should have been on top of the world. Instead, I was packing my bags for rehab, not quite understanding how I had let it get this bad.

I felt I owed it to my employer to let them in on what was going on. I was nervous and resisted the urge to come clean at first. They would no doubt be disappointed. *Will I lose my starting job? Will the media catch wind of this? More importantly, will the front office take away my newly signed $30-million deal?* I didn't care. I was broken and had hit rock bottom. My family and my health were more important.

Most guys in their early 30s don't really care that much about their health. Maybe they, too, feel like they're invincible. But my family has a history of heart trouble, high blood pressure, you name it. Here I was, playing Russian roulette with 60, sometimes 100 milligrams of Adderall, not understanding what it was doing to my long-term health. I knew I couldn't control the drug. It definitely was controlling me. And that scared the hell out of me. I had to stick around for my kids. See them grow up, not check out permanently like my dad had done at age 30.

I called Bruce Bochy. Bruce had always shot straight with me, and I respected the hell out of the guy. Sometimes after games, Pat and I would go in and hang out in his office and shoot the breeze with him...talk about the season...how we thought everyone was doing in the clubhouse. It was definitely the first time I had experienced that on any team; and in my opinion, Bruce was the number one reason we won the championship.

He was the kind of man's man that I looked up to and desperately wanted to be. In a way he was everything I had hoped my father would have been. Bruce is currently a three-time World Series winning manager on his way to Cooperstown, but you wouldn't know it by his confident, yet humble, demeanor.

He treated every player on the team with an utmost respect and confidence in their ability to get the job done. He was a pro at managing all sorts of personalities, a skill definitely required with our club of characters, and one not many other managers around the league possess.

I felt like he loved Pat and me like his own sons, and he cared about us as guys, not just our on-field performance. I knew he could be trusted and would not let anyone else know about my secret, so I shot straight with him. I came clean and laid it all out on the table, confessing not only what I had done recently, but also what I did off the field all last season as my drinking and partying raged out of control. He was shocked and saddened to hear about all that I had gone through. I felt like he had my back. And it felt amazing to let it all out.

At the end of the call I'll never forget what he said. "Aubrey, I really had no idea things were going that bad for you off the field. All I know is that you were truly an inspiration last year, not only on the field but in the clubhouse as one of my leaders. If it weren't for you, there's no way in hell we would have won this thing. But I know how much more important family and your health are. Please get done what you need to get done, and let's get you back ready to make a run at another title." He never mentioned a word to anyone, true to his character.

I zipped up my luggage and dragged it out to the curb as I cast a last look over my shoulder at my lonely hotel apartment. I felt scared and dejected as I sat in the back of a cab headed to the airport, hurtling toward an unknown future. I sat there replaying the scene from just a couple of months prior in my head.

As the film rolled in my head, I saw a picturesque midmorning day in San Francisco. November 3rd, to be exact. I was one of the lucky few players to be chosen to address the crowd at our official celebration in downtown San Francisco to celebrate the 2010 championship season. I'd be speaking in front of over 1,000,000 grateful, diehard Giants fans.

Each player shared a personal cable car with one other teammate and their families. My partner for the ride that day obviously was Pat. This was our first parade, but you wouldn't have known it. He and I were the only players who had planned ahead for the two-hour ride through the narrow, winding streets, through Market Street toward downtown. Our cable car was equipped with our own personal cooler, stocked with a case of ice-cold Bud Lights. Pat and I enjoyed the atmosphere, sipping back ice-cold brews, relishing the adoration of the fans with our families in tow. Orange and black confetti fell all around us. The smell of marijuana from the free-spirited crowd filled the air at every turn.

As usual, the beers were going down like water. I never thought to look for a bathroom on the cable car when I boarded, and now my bladder was at max capacity. I had to pee so bad I could taste it. I checked both ends of the cable car, and to my horror found nowhere to take a leak! I seriously thought about just pissing my pants right there and then, but decided against it. Standing at a podium on live TV with a huge urine stain down the front of my pants seemed like a bad idea, no matter how many beers I had in me. The only bathrooms in sight were nasty portable ones at the end of each block. Getting to them meant navigating an infinite sea of rabid Giants fans. I couldn't do that. I'd get ambushed. I had only one option.

I made my way to the back of the car and got into push-up position, just below the sight line of the fans. I unzipped my pants and let it flow all over the floor of the moving cable car. My wife was appalled. Jayce thought it was hilarious as a hot stream of urine began to rush under his feet. I didn't even flinch as I got up, zipped back up, and grabbed another beer. My degeneracy knew no limits.

We finally arrived at our final destination right smack in the middle of downtown. City hall. After the governor of California, Arnold Schwarzenegger, addressed the crowd and congratulated the team, it was the players' turn to acknowledge what were truly the best fans in all of baseball. You could tell it had been a long time since anyone had lifted a trophy in that city. It seemed like everyone and his dog were out that day.

Knowing what I had planned for my speech, many of my teammates knew I'd be a tough act to follow, so I agreed to go last. After Buster Posey finished his final words, it was now my turn to approach the podium. I wasn't nervous at all. 40 milligrams and many quarts of Bud Light made sure I felt like a real celebrity for the first time in my life. The sense of power and invincibility I felt while up at that podium was intoxicating. I was digging the adoration to say the least. But a speech was not all I had in mind that day. I thought it to be a good idea to surprise the fans of San

Francisco with a little comic relief. Something to remember the team by.

My red "rally thong" had become a symbol for our team chock-full of misfits and castoffs from other organizations. I had never been a part of such an amazing group of teammates. We came from all walks of life, but couldn't be more alike. We had a great cast of veteran leadership that started with guys like Matt Cain, Edgar Renteria, Jeremy Affeldt, Javier Lopez, Barry Zito, Freddy Sanchez, Mark Derosa, Aaron Rowand, Andres Torres, Juan Uribe, Nate Schierholtz, and Cody Ross. We had the young studs like Buster Posey, Madison Bumgarner, and Tim Lincecum, whose talent matched their maturity. Then we had some real nuts added in there for good measure. Of course Pat, Brian Wilson and I rounded out that group.

I wound up my rambling speech, thanking the fans for their undying support all season. Now it was time for my alter ego, Huffdaddy, to make his appearance. With my red thong already stuffed down my pants, I was ready for action. In the movie *Zoolander*, there is a scene in which Derek Zoolander, played by Ben Stiller has a runway model walk off with arch rival Hansel, played by Owen Wilson. At the end of the walk off, Hansel pulls out his underwear without ever taking off his pants, waving it above his head. This is the scene I was inspired to recreate in front of a million Giants fans and millions more on live TV.

I ended my speech with, "And now, if you have seen the movie *Zoolander*, I have a special talent just for you." I moved to the side of the podium confidently so the whole crowd could see. I reached down into my pants with my right hand, moving my hips violently, getting ready to "remove" my red-and-black rally thong without taking off my pants. I pulled it out, and raised it proudly above my head, stretching it out with both hands nice and high for all to see. The crowd erupted in applause and laughter. My teammates laughed uncontrollably, as one of my favorite teammates of all time, Andres Torres came racing over to give me a high five. My hands had been down my pants just a second earlier, but he didn't care. We were truly the tightest band of brothers I had ever played with. I couldn't see my wife. She was no doubt crouched low, hiding herself in embarrassment somewhere in the crowd. Search YouTube for "Aubrey Huff rally thong" to get a better visual.

Confetti rained down on us from high above city hall. A fitting end to a season full of personal degeneracy off the field. And a culmination of all I had worked hard for my whole life on the field.

As special and funny as that moment was, I couldn't help but think of how Adderall was messing with my decision-making. Adderall transformed me from a shy, awkward kid from Texas with no confidence whatsoever to Huffdaddy, a guy not afraid to pull out women's underwear from his pants in front of an entire city. On Adderall I did things I never in a million years would have done clean.

I sank back into the backseat of the cab. I really had no idea what the next 30-plus days would be like for me.

Russ had agreed to pick me up from the Scottsdale airport and give me a ride to the facility. I can't say I enjoyed our conversation during the 45-minute drive to the facility. I was Adderall-free that day for the first time in a long time. My head was already beginning to go dark and blank, and my energy level was moderate at best. Russ and I spoke of our friendship. Of better days. And how much better the days would be once again, after rehab.

Russ knew me better than anyone. After all, he was my best man at my wedding. He had been there for me for the good and the bad. He drove slowly in the right-hand lane, as if he wanted to stretch the ride out. He said to me softly, "I'm so proud you're doing this, buddy. Baubi and I chatted the other day over the phone, and we both know this is something you must do or you're going to end up losing everything."

I had no idea they had chatted, and I responded, "Did you get a sense from her that she would take me back after this?"

Russ answered, "It's not going to hurt your cause."

Thoughts began flooding my mind as we got closer to Sundance. *Will she take me back? Will this just be a big waste of time? It's only Adderall. I don't have a drug problem! I could actually use an Adderall right now, as a matter of fact!* As my doubt and anxiousness grew, I said to Russ, "Buddy, I don't need to go to rehab, I can quit right now. Let's just turn this car around and go back, I can beat this cold turkey!"

He immediately pulled the car over to the side of the road just blocks away from our destination. He threw it into park violently, looking me dead in the eye with all seriousness and said, "Aubrey, if you don't complete this rehab, not only will you lose your wife and kids, but you'll also lose a best friend. Do you understand?" I had never seen him so serious in all the years I had known him. I nodded in unconvincing agreement.

We pulled into the Sundance driveway. I couldn't have felt more embarrassed and ashamed. I was still on the fence, not knowing if I really needed help. The left side of my brain reasoned that I was just using Adderall, a prescription drug that people were using all over the world. *Maybe I do have ADHD. Maybe I really do need this stuff.* I was convinced the other guys at Sundance were strung out on coke, heroin, or worse. Real drugs! *They are going to think I'm crazy for even being here.*

Russ interrupted my train of thought. "I love ya, buddy, and I know you're going to kick this addiction. See you in no time." He hugged me and walked back to his car. He drove away never looking back as I fought back tears. I wanted to get my family back. I had to get through this hell.

I hesitantly walked through the front door, dragging with me a negative attitude. *I don't need to be here*, I thought as I began to look around to take in my surroundings for the next month and a half. In my experience, nobody and no amount of rehab can help you if you don't want to change. You have to desperately want it for yourself. You have to have a desperate need for change. I wasn't sure I *wanted* to change. I liked not being the real me. The real me had no idea how to be a confident man. As a matter of fact just seconds after walking through that door I couldn't help but think about the first day of spring training. There, I could get a fresh bottle of black-and-orange pills. Feel like a real man again.

I was met by one of the counselors who introduced me to everyone on staff. Everyone seemed nice enough. Now it was time to meet the patients. The cast of characters was just as I pictured it would be. There was a 60 year-old man who had consumed a bottle of vodka a day since he was eighteen. There was a 15 year-old boy who was hooked on heroin, needle marks all up and down his arms. There was a 30 year-old woman hooked up to an oxygen tank, looking like she was 65. The majority of the addicts there were tattoo-covered, speed and cocaine junkies who looked like they were straight off the streets. Rounding out the group were several normal-looking prescription-pill addicts just like me.

Why am I here? This is so embarrassing. I don't have a problem. It's just pills. Prescription meds given to kids. Not real drugs like heroin or cocaine. I could imagine myself sitting in a circle as everyone introduced themselves... "Hi, I'm James, I am addicted to heroin. Hi, I'm Jane, and I'm addicted to cocaine." Then, it would be my turn. "Hi, I'm Aubrey. Um. I take Adderall."

The first week without Adderall or booze in my system was absolute misery. I never thought I could feel so depressed, worthless, and tired all the time. I always wondered how someone could ever get so low that they would actually think about killing themselves. Well now I finally understood. I was so irritable and mean to whomever I came across. I know I wasn't making any friends there, that's for sure, and quite frankly, I didn't want to.

I was only there for a couple of days before everybody found out I had just won a World Series. I was sure they thought I was just a self-righteous prick. I was absolutely dying for a pill! The headaches were unbearable, as were the aches and pains from my shoulders all the way down to my ankles that Adderall must have been masking for months. Now that I no longer had that crutch to lean on, I felt like I was in a living hell.

I had heard numerous horror stories of people who had to detox drugs out of their system. I didn't truly understand it until I had to go through it myself. The argument I had made earlier about Adderall not being a real drug was obviously hogwash. Whatever was leaving my system as I detoxed that first week was obviously a real drug. I found myself sweating profusely and freezing at the same time most nights. I tried desperately to get the sleep my body craved, but I just rolled from one side to the other trying to get comfortable. The only time I could fall asleep was when I cried uncontrollably until my body and emotions decompressed from a lifetime of pent-up fear and selfishness.

I boarded the bus to the gym twice a week. But I did not go to work out. It was basically my only escape from the prison. Like a guy doing hard time who jumps at the chance to do roadside cleanup just for a change of scenery for a few hours.

Spring training was literally just around the corner now, and I was in absolutely no physical or mental condition to begin the grind of a 162-game season. I started to wonder what kind of player I would be without Adderall. Would these aches and pains go away eventually? Would I ever get myself back to a sense of normalcy mentally? Would I be as good offensively as I was last year? I had serious doubts about all these questions, and more.

I began to panic about not being in shape going into the season. I hadn't hit a weight or picked up a bat in months. I tried to get something started at the gym, but I just didn't have the energy to do more than twenty minutes on the treadmill each time. The very thought of a real workout made me want to puke.

While on Adderall, I literally had to remind myself to eat something every few hours. It killed my appetite. Now I ate everything in sight. Eating was an escape from my depressed state if only for a little while. Surprisingly, the food at Sundance was quite good, and it was there waiting for me any time I felt like a meal. This, combined with weeks of zero physical activity, had me quickly gaining 15 pounds, right in the love handles and gut.

I settled in and went about the assignments Sundance organized for us to keep us busy. I was just going through the motions though. I committed to doing just the bare minimum, never participating in group, and only doing a half-ass job on my assignments, just enough to scrape by. My negative attitude upon arrival now grew into an attitude of defiance. The only thing I looked forward to twice a week were my hour-long sessions with a therapist named Annette.

Annette was a tough-nosed, no-nonsense type of woman. She had a tough mentality about her and wasn't afraid to drop some curse words to get her point across. She reminded me of many of the teammates I had played with in years past. She wouldn't fall for any of my fake macho facade and saw right through my phony act. With that kind of attitude, she quickly earned my respect. She made it her mission to break me, and one day she did.

We began our session talking about whether I thought my stay at Sundance was helping. We talked about my wife and kids, and what I could do to help them trust me again. We talked about playing baseball sober, and what I could do mentally to maintain my edge without drugs. But the real breakthrough came when she began digging into my relationship with my father, or lack thereof. I told her how my father was murdered when I was six, and how I never really knew him. She asked me, "Did you love him?"

I was taken aback because I had never asked myself that question. Confused, I replied, "Well, it should be a simple yes, but he was never there for any of us. The only real image I have of him was sitting in a recliner with a beer in hand, completely ignoring us. So I guess the answer would be no."

She continued, "How does that vision of your dad make you feel today?"

A desperate angry sadness crept in, and I began getting edgy. I pinched up. "It pisses me off, to be honest with you, Annette! How could he have done this to me? I never really learned how to be a man, and I needed him to show me how. Now I'm nothing but a scared little boy who ended up in *this* hellhole! I always seem to be afraid, like I don't stack up to other guys." My eyes welled up with tears.

It was then I realized I had been harboring a genuine disdain for my father for a long time. I wanted to love him, but I just couldn't. After all, I never really knew him. I don't even remember the sound of his voice. Annette leaned into me, eye to eye, and with a very stern face said, "Aubrey, you don't want to be that father to *your* boys, do you?"

I lost it. I cried like there was no tomorrow as the reality of that question hit me right between the eyes. I knew right then and there what was happening to me. I was turning into my father. I was becoming his mirror image. Ignoring my kids just as he had me. Even if Baubi divorced me after this, I still needed to be a dad. I had to be a dad for my boys!

Annette's question woke me up that afternoon. I made it my number one priority in life right then and there to be the best dad I possibly could. But first I had to get sober!

Rehab was a very confusing time for me. Days dragged on forever. Every day I was sober, I remembered a new low that I had desperately tried to forget. I spent most of my time in my room in absolute silence with nothing but my thoughts. Bored out of my mind. But my time there was about to get really interesting.

The Bible tells great stories of God communicating with humans while they wander alone in the desert. Well, ironically enough, I was in the desert, finally sober and quiet enough to hear him whisper to me one evening.

Each day just before sunset, most patients would be outside smoking cigarettes and drinking coffee over by a very large putting green. We would all hang out and chat before our final group session of the day. A few of us would attempt to make the 60-foot putt through small rolling hills that would be almost impossible to make even for a pro golfer. We had been trying every day for weeks now, without any luck.

One of the facility therapists came out to call us in for our session. The sun was beginning to set, putting off picturesque pinks and purples across the beautiful, partly cloudy desert horizon. A few guys stirred, and eventually, everyone headed inside for what was sure to be yet another long and boring session. I stayed put, however. I sat down in a chair next to the putting green with a putter in hand contemplating whether to even go in. I was bitter and confused. I was going through another one of those cycles, seriously wondering what was so bad about Adderall after all. I knew it made me feel good and enhanced every activity I immersed myself in. I knew it made me feel invincible on the baseball field. I was feeling pretty disgusted that I even had to be in rehab.

Then, the other side of the cycle started. Perhaps the logical part of my mind kicked in. *On the other hand,* I thought, *Adderall was turning me into an unfaithful husband and an uninvolved father.*

Being drug-free was definitely a step in the right direction. I felt that. But, I was not convinced that I could magically become a good father and husband. Something was missing. I knew I could be better. Do better. I just had no idea how to get there. I was desperate for some answers.

I felt overwhelmed with emotion. What had become of my life? Why was I so emotionally detached when I had achieved all this success? Why was there this huge hole in my heart?

Rehab was hardly the place I expected God to come knocking. I definitely don't feel like I deserved his attention. Nor was I listening for it. But he did. I heard God speak to me loud and clear that evening. Not something audible, just an incredibly overwhelming feeling in my heart that was hard to deny. I knew the feeling wasn't coming from me.

"Aubrey, pray to me. I still love you."

Where had this unexpected thought come from? I hadn't thought of God in ages! I was sort of mad at God at this time in my life, and certainly didn't feel like he was particularly concerned about me.

I looked around and saw no one. Everyone else was inside the building. The sky was on fire. Absolutely beautiful. Like one of those sunsets that you can't even photograph because it just wouldn't do it justice.

It had been so long since I prayed, I wasn't even sure that God existed anymore. I had my doubts that what I heard was anything but a random thought. So as a joke really, I bowed my head, and almost as a challenge, prayed out loud, "Lord, if that was really you, or if you even exist, please let me know somehow. Please just give me a sign." As I sat there in the chair, putter still in hand, I upped the ante. "I tell you what, God, if I make this putt, I'll know that you're really there and that you really love me."

I stood up, picked up a golf ball lying close by and set it down at the very edge of the green, a full 60 feet away from the cup. I looked around again. Not a soul in sight. Strangely, I felt like I wasn't alone. I didn't take the time to square up the shot or aim all that much, I just gently swung the cheap putter and hit the ball. I watched it roll down the green at what I felt was a good speed, but not necessarily on a great path. It headed toward the edge of the green, like it had done dozens of other times for me before. All of a sudden, the ball hit the side of one of the small, hill-like bumps and took a hard right. Now it was heading right toward the hole, but ever so slowly. *Not enough speed to make it,* I thought. But out of the blue, the ball picked up speed, almost like it caught another gear. Straight for the cup. It went in!

I immediately got chills from head to toe; even now as I type this, I'm feeling those chills once again. I walked the length of the green some 25 strides away to retrieve the ball from the cup, laughing, thinking what a coincidence it was. I mean, what were the odds? I reached down to grab the ball and brought it up for a closer look. My breath literally left my body as I stood there staring, trying to wrap my mind around what I was seeing. You know how Callaway golf balls have numbers on them? Either a 1, 2, 3, or 4 so you can identify your ball? Well, this particular ball happened to be a 4. But it was an old ball that been hit so much that the black ink on the number 4 had started to wear off. As I held it with what would be the number 4 facing me upside down, I noticed the diagonal part of the number had worn off, making it look exactly like a cross! That ball sits in a glass case in my man cave to this day. It is my most prized possession. Far more valuable than any autographed guitar, movie memorabilia, or baseball artifact in my huge collection. I even value that ball more than my two World Series rings.

I asked God for a sign, and I think he gave it.

I was amazed at what had happened that night. I shared the story with the group, showing each of them the ball. I held on to it the whole time, making sure I didn't lose it.

Any regular guy given these circumstances would have immediately gotten on the straight and narrow. But not Aubrey Huff III.

The same old thoughts flooded back the next day. *I just have to make it through this crap so I can get back at what I do best.* My rehab stint was to end just a few days after spring training started, but the idea of missing even a single day of the action was driving me absolutely nuts. So I made up a little white lie.

According to my fictional tale, a San Francisco beat writer had called me, asking me if it was indeed true that I was at a rehab facility. I went on to explain to the staff that I felt like a flood of reporters could show up at the facility any day now. I didn't want to be found out, or make the other patients uncomfortable. They bought the lie, and agreed to release me a few days early. My wife fell for it, too.

As an addict and a drunk, I developed an uncanny ability to lie without any sense of remorse whatsoever. The lying fed off itself. It got so bad in fact that I began to believe my own lies. Things I lied about honestly felt like they actually happened. A very scary place to be.

Mark Twain said, "If you tell the truth, you don't have to remember anything."

I had to remember a lot.

CHAPTER FOURTEEN
7-ELEVEN

*"I planned to relapse
the second I walked out of
that place."*

—Eminem

I'd checked the box. Rehab completed. Baubi *had* to take me back now. But she and the boys wouldn't be joining me until the start of the regular season a month and a half later. I rented a small house in North Scottsdale, Arizona, far away from the Old Town party scene that was sure to be calling my name. I wanted to be as far away from that as possible so I could focus on the task at hand...getting ready for the new season.

Baubi had given me the chance I had asked for, but it came with a price. She told me over the phone that she would personally be doing random drug tests at any time, any place she felt appropriate. I was just glad to have Jayce and Jagger back, and at this point didn't care what strings were attached.

But now came the real test. I would be solo for the next 45 days, back in the same environment I was so accustomed to using in. I had my doubts I would be able to stay strong. Part of me knew I had a free pass to use until the start of the season when Baubi and the kids would join me back in San Francisco. But I also knew that if I started using again, I wouldn't be able to stop.

I was determined to stay clean. To not blow the chance. I had no idea how in the world I was ever going to replace the Adderall-infused invincibility I had enjoyed the season before, and I must say reporting back to spring camp felt awkward. It was good to see the guys again, but I wondered if somehow some of the guys found out but didn't want to say anything about my stint at Sundance. Not even Bruce Bochy said a word about it. It was as if it had never happened.

I should have been excited to be back, ready to defend the World Series title, but I was very sullen. I felt so naked, insecure, and uninspired walking to my locker without my morning pill. My mind was already yearning for the little orange-and-white pill that had become my best friend. It was hard to resist the urge to reach for the bottle right before we hit the field for our very first practice, but I knew I couldn't blow it on the first day back. I found myself having to trick my mind, trying to convince myself that I was excited to take the field. But reality set in the minute I stepped out onto the field.

Practice was an absolute bore! I couldn't focus. My mind wandered to the million other places I would rather have been. My killer instinct was gone. So were my excitement, passion, and determination. I felt like a zombie going through the monotonous drills the typical spring training day entails. *Like getting teeth pulled at the dentist*, I thought. Torture!

Even the diehard Giants fans I had fallen in love with the previous season were annoying the hell out of me. I thought to myself, *Don't these morons have anything better to do on a random Tuesday than to waste time watching batting practice?*

To make matters worse, the pain in my lower back from all the standing around was really beginning to bother me, and I felt like I had the energy level of a sloth. *There is no way I can make it a whole season like this.* The preseason was just a few hours old and I already knew I would either have to use or remain a zombie. Be the player I was last year or hang on to my wife and children and risk losing my starting job. Then a thought came to me. *Maybe I don't have to choose. Maybe I can have both!*

Surely the drug tests Baubi would be administering would be the urine type. There was no way she could do the blood testing that the MLB does. A light bulb went off in my head. Maybe, just maybe, I could convince someone to supply me with a clean source of urine in time for my family's arrival in San Francisco for opening day.

My attitude changed as I realized I had a shot to use with no strings attached that entire spring. The next morning couldn't come soon enough!

It had been almost two months since the Adderall had detoxed out of my system, and I was ready to feel alive again. I awoke with a renewed sense of excitement as I jumped out of bed and headed to the kitchen. I knew my appetite would be gone after popping a pill, so I made sure to eat a big breakfast before heading out...an egg-white omelet and some oatmeal.

I hopped into my Lexus GS 430 with a heavy foot, easily doing 95 headed south on Highway 101 to Scottsdale Stadium right in the heart of Old Town.

Screeching to a halt in the players' lot, I practically ran into the clubhouse, straight for the training room, ignoring the hordes of fans screaming for autographs just outside our clubhouse entrance. *I have to collect my monthly Adderall script.*

The drug addict in me sprang to life. I was shaking as I struggled to get the white cap off the orange bottle as fast as possible. I downed a 20-milligram pill, my first in months, before I even made it out of the training room. I chased it down with someone else's half-empty coffee.

I sat at my locker waiting for the effect to kick in. An overwhelming sense of guilt washed over me. *What the hell is wrong with me?* Just a day earlier I had felt so determined to play the season clean. It had taken me less than 24 hours to do a complete one-eighty and betray the trust my wife had placed in me. My mind took me back to the golf ball incident. I pushed the feelings of guilt out of my mind, choosing to forget about my children and God. All the counseling, the crap I put up with in "'prison"' at Sundance...none of it mattered now. The guilt splintered my mind. I sat there patiently, knowing the guilt would soon be replaced by confidence and excitement. And for that I was willing to sacrifice anything.

Sure enough, the sensation hit me like a wave. The Huffdaddy of last season was back! I was confident, talkative, carefree, energetic, excited, sure of myself, and ready to lead this team to back-to-back World Series titles.

The Adderall-fueled-me became one of the league leaders in home runs and batting average that spring. It was easily the best spring I had ever had. I was amped and ready to get off to a hot start back in California.

But before we broke camp for the West Coast, I had to find a reliable source of clean urine for the season. Asking someone in the clubhouse obviously wasn't an option. I had a sudden flash of brilliance. I knew just who to ask. Roger, a die-hard Giants fan that lived just two doors down from me, would surely help me out. I should have been nervous ringing his doorbell that afternoon but Adderall took any hesitation away. I can only imagine what was going through his mind as I explained my situation and asked him to pee in a bottle. I am just so glad he agreed.

I handed him an empty water bottle immediately and said, "Take a leak in it for me, and fill it all the way to the top for the flight home. Baubi will be there when I arrive, and you never know, she may just have a test ready."

I was pumped and ready to take on the 2011 season as we left Scottsdale in the rearview mirror. I had finished the 2010 season seventh in the National League's Most Valuable Player Award voting. My goal was to actually be the MVP that season. I was convinced I could do it, especially if I kept hitting the ball like I had been all spring.

Baubi had found a nice rental in Hillsborough, 20 minutes away from AT&T Park. It felt amazing to have my family back. I pushed the fact I had lied to them and had been using all spring out of my mind. All seemed right with the world. My only worry now was hoping my plan would help me pass Baubi's random drug tests.

One of the first things I did when I walked into our rental home was to hide the contraband in the master bathroom right in that little space behind the toilet where nobody ever looks or cleans.

I hadn't even unpacked my suitcase when Baubi appeared behind me in my closet with a testing kit for amphetamines in hand. She stood there with a standard Walgreens-issue urine test, ready for a sample.

"No problem, baby," I said as I walked calmly to the master bathroom. I locked the door behind me and filled the cup with the clean urine. I passed. *I will need way more than one bottle to get me through this season,* I thought. I needed to find a San Francisco urine supplier, and I knew just the guy.

I had met Derrick at a restaurant he managed on Market Street the year prior, and struck up a good friendship with him. We had even hung out at his house from time to time. He too was a die-hard Giants fan, a fitness nut, and I knew for a fact he didn't even drink. He would be perfect!

As luck would have it, Derrick lived off the same exit I did in Hillsboro. I'll spare you the details. Just know that Derrick supplied me with more than enough clean urine than I needed all season. Problem solved!

To my absolute shock, I struggled mightily the first month of the season. The magic from the spring was gone. I was into the game, but something else was occupying my mind. An overwhelming sense of guilt haunted me. Even though I was high 24/7, I just couldn't shake the heaviness that came with using behind Baubi's back.

I was 35 and felt convinced that if I just kept using Adderall for just another three years, I could retire and be done with it forever. Playing without it was simply not an option at this point.

The league didn't care; I still had my TUE. My fear was that I would get caught using by Baubi. The paranoia built, and all I could think about each morning after popping my pill was that this could be the day I would fail the test and lose it all.

I was still struggling at the plate two months later all because my mind continued to torment me. Miraculously, I had passed numerous random drug tests from Baubi, but the crushing guilt that was deep in my conscience was at a tipping point. Something had to give. A big part of me just wanted to be honest with my wife. But I knew if I did that she would definitely leave me. And to be honest, that started sounding like a viable plan in the state I was in. At least then I could finish out my baseball career without having to answer to anybody!

But I couldn't lose Jayce and Jagger! I knew I would never make it without them in my life. Even though I wasn't necessarily about to earn Father of the Year, I really enjoyed seeing their smiling faces every day. Even though I never really showed it, I loved them more than anything on the planet. I knew that one day I would be done with baseball and be able to be the father they deserve.

Now, years later, I realize I am not the only guy who struggled with balancing work and home life. I know so many guys today who seem to have to make a choice between a career and a family. Finding the right balance is definitely not an easy task.

Why can't the Adderall burn through all this guilt? I thought. *I mean I didn't suffer from any guilt last season!* Then it hit me. *It has to be the golf ball experience with God at rehab.* Since that moment, I had known that God was trying to get my attention and was more than willing to help me clean up my act and become the man I knew deep down I could be. I realized that even before I would pop my pill every morning, it wasn't necessarily my wife and kids that were the first to pop in my mind making me feel guilty. It was God!

I had to get rid of that nagging Godly guilt. The guilt had to go! It was then that I decided God was dead. As far as I was concerned at that time, God never existed in the first place. It was an easy choice to make given the mental state I was in. I felt better almost immediately. The guilt lifted, and I was again able to focus on the most important person in the world at the time. Me.

June 2nd rolled around, and we were playing the St. Louis Cardinals at Busch Stadium in St. Louis. I was beginning to heat up at the plate a bit, and felt my game improving tremendously now that I had shed the God guilt baggage. That day was magical. I had my first-ever three-home-run game! It was an incredible feeling.

When I was a kid, I watched one of my childhood Texas Rangers idols, Juan Gonzalez, hit three home runs in one game. I always thought that would be a cool thing to do. It just so happened that my wife's birthday fell on that particular day, June 2nd. The perfect day to be recognized as the player of the game.

I was asked to do a post-game interview for *CSN Bay Area* with Mike Krukow and Duane Kuiper, longtime, legendary broadcasters for the Giants. "Kuip," as players affectionately called him, asked me, "Aubrey, how does your first-ever three-home-run game feel?"

Jittery from the Adderall and the excitement of the game, I responded, "It feels amazing, that's one of the things I had always wanted to do in my big league career was to have a three-home-run game. Kind of ironic it just so happened to fall on my wife's birthday." I pointed my finger toward the camera and continued, "Those homers were for you, baby!" Here I was dedicating that game during a post-game interview to my wife for her birthday. High as a kite. Deceiving her like I had been the whole season.

As we touched down at the airport in San Francisco, I had to make a quick stop at Derrick's house to pick up a fresh bottle of urine he had left sitting in his mailbox for me. I finally walked into our house around one a.m. Everyone was asleep. I passed out, exhausted.

I awoke around noon the next day, eyes still blurry from another restless night's sleep. My eyes began to focus enough to notice I had a drug test sitting on my bedside table waiting for me. Suddenly I realized I had left my urine bottle in the car out in the garage the night before. My heart began to race. In order to get to the garage, I had to walk through the kitchen. Baubi was already up with the boys. If she saw me walk out there, she'd know something was up. I had to think of something, and fast!

So instead of heading through the kitchen, I crept out the back door into the back yard as quietly as I could. I hopped over the fence and crouched low, entering the garage through the small door in the back. I was so glad it wasn't locked! I frantically searched under the passenger seat of my car and grabbed the bottle, scurrying back over the fence and back to the master bedroom. I have no idea how I made it undetected. In the bathroom, I filled the cup up from the bottle like I had done so many times before, and placed it back on the bedside table. Piece of cake!

I began to get angry as I walked down the hallway to join my family in the living room. *I mean, this is starting to piss me off. How many more damn tests do I have to pass before this woman trusts me again? Uncle!*

I waltzed into the living room and gave each of my boys a kiss good morning. Baubi didn't even acknowledge me. She disappeared into the bedroom, no doubt checking on my sample. She knew I was using. She just couldn't prove it. And the cat-and-mouse game was really starting to get to her, too.

She came back into the living room a few minutes later, looked at me sternly, and motioned, "follow me." I followed her down the hallway to the master bedroom, thoughts dancing in my head. *What did I do wrong? Did I fail the test? Is Derrick using too?*

She picked up the sample cup and held it within a foot of my face. Her voice trembling, ready to explode, she asked, "Why in the hell is this urine sample 75 degrees on the temperature strip? Does your piss run cold like your heart?"

I had never noticed the temperature strips on the sides of the testing cups. She hadn't either until now. A fresh sample runs in the 90- to 100-degree range. *How am I going to get myself out of this jam?*

I got defensive. "Well, I did pee in that cup like 30 minutes ago. Probably doesn't take too long for urine to get to room temperature."

She screamed, "You're lucky I don't have another test right now or I'd make you pee in it right in front of me. I don't believe you! I know you have been using, and this proves it! I'm going to Walgreens right now, you prick!"

I panicked, as I yelled back, "You go ahead and go to Walgreens. I'll take the test when I get home! I'm not waiting around here for you. I have to get to the yard and make a living for us!" I turned and walked toward my closet. Just then, Baubi reached out and grabbed my arm, pulling me back to her. I turned to look her in the eye. The look she gave me was of pure madness. "You aren't going anywhere until I get back, do you understand me?"

I lost it. At that moment, I turned into someone I did not recognize. Someone I am still afraid of today. Someone who is not rational, and quite frankly, dangerous. I grabbed Baubi by the throat and slammed her up against the closet wall. Something in my mind wanted to go further, but I fought the urge. I let go, immediately regretting what I had done.

The look in her eyes was of genuine fear. I was scared, too. *What kind of a monster have I become? How could I hurt my wife? The mother of my kids? Someone I am supposed to love?* She ran out of the closet crying.

I got dressed and headed to the field.

I decided we needed a breather so I stayed in a hotel downtown after the game that night. Thankfully, Baubi had previously planned a trip to Westlake Village, California, the next day to look at some possible homes. A place to retire to after I hung up my cleats. Funny how that future was looking ever so dim now.

Now I had this stupid temperature strip to deal with, I had to craft a new plan. How could I keep the clean sample warm enough each night? And what if she decided to test me in the morning? It's not like I could keep the urine at 95 degrees 24/7 waiting for a test.

I crafted what I thought was a cunning plan. I would pull into the 7-Eleven on the way home from work each night. The store was just three miles from our house. I would pull out one of the bottles I kept stashed in my trunk and zap it in the microwave for a few seconds. It wasn't a perfect science, but I figured 15 seconds should do the job. If she didn't test me that night, I'd just stash the bottle under the bathroom sink and run hot water over it long enough to pass a test.

Even with all my deceptive plans and the anger toward my wife, I was unaware I had a problem. In the state I was in, I honestly thought that I wasn't harming anybody.

On the field, however, there was plenty of harm surrounding the entire team. On June 10th, veteran second baseman Freddy Sanchez dislocated his shoulder diving for a ground ball. He would go on to have season-ending surgery. On May 25th in extra innings, Florida Marlins utility man Scott Cousins collided with Buster Posey, fracturing Buster's ankle, also ending his season. On July 15th, Pat Burrell was placed on the disabled list with a foot injury. An injury that basically ended his career. Cody Ross's calf and hamstring issues kept him hampered all season. And to top it all off, our All Star closer, Brian Wilson, was shut down in August due to inflammation in his pitching elbow.

Five serious injuries. I basically watched as our 2011 season was flushed down the toilet. Suddenly, all the offensive pressure was on me. Remember, I had just signed that big three-year, $30-million deal. I was now the guy everyone was looking to. And when I wasn't able to carry the load offensively, I naturally became the whipping boy. My lack of preparation during the offseason was now showing up as a real lack of production. I fast became a huge disappointment.

The pressure to perform mounted. I had to blame someone or something for my lack of delivery. And it sure wasn't about to be me! I thought to myself, *If Baubi didn't make me go to rehab, I wouldn't be having this bad of a season. Not to mention all the damn drug tests she's making me take. It's driving me crazy!* I started to truly resent and dislike my wife for putting me in such a situation. I didn't stop for a second to consider my role in all of it.

Looking back on it now, I was such a douchebag. I wasn't a man. I wasn't a husband or father. I don't know what I was. I guess you could say I was a liar, a coward, a scumbag, a drunk, an abusive husband, an addict...the list goes on and on.

The resentment toward Baubi allowed me to justify staying out even later. I stayed out late even when we played at home. I disengaged and withdrew from my family. I didn't cook, clean, or help with the kids. All I did every day was use, go play ball, and drink until I passed out. Baubi and I never spoke. And the only interaction I had with my kids was when I would sit to watch TV with them. Sometimes I would read them a book before I would put them to bed when we had a day game, but I would read the book super-fast and slam it shut. I'd get it over with so I could go outside to have a beer and a smoke. I had turned into my father, and in a weird way I was okay with that.

The season was coming to a close, and it was obvious that we weren't going to make the playoffs. My playing time was starting to dwindle, however, the frequency of the drug tests at home was increasing. Who could blame Baubi? My behavior was definitely not that of a normal guy's. The cat-and-mouse game continued. It's truly amazing to me that my wife never caught me red-handed.

I had no doubt in my mind that if I failed a single test, she would be gone in an instant. The kids were the only reason she stayed anyhow. She was repulsed by me, and believe me, I could tell.

Baubi was solid as a rock that season. I couldn't help but notice how at peace she was with the children. She had truly become a wonderful mom. Yes, I was driving her absolutely insane, but that did not deter her from being the parent our boys needed in their crucial infant and toddler years. She did it all with zero help from me, and did an amazing job.

I watched the way Jayce and Jagger would gravitate toward her in any situation. When we were both in the room, it was always about Mom. They wanted nothing to do with me. It was a very lonely, sickening, depressing feeling. My own two boys were supposed to be all about their daddy, but they wanted nothing to do with me. Who could blame them? Now, I not only resented Baubi, I was jealous, too.

About the only production happening so far that season was Derrick's urine supply. I had been steadily building up my clean urine supply in preparation for the offseason, and now had a personal stash of almost a dozen bottles with just a few weeks of the season remaining.

We finished the year at 86-76, second place in the National League West, obviously missing the playoffs. The season was over, and I breathed a huge sigh of relief. I was glad we didn't make the playoffs. The testing at home was driving me insane.

Driving home after the final game of the season, a fresh bottle of urine laying in the seat next to me, I thought, *Damn. I'm actually going to get away with using all year. This urine idea actually worked!*

I pulled into the 7-Eleven to warm up the urine bottle one last time.

I strolled into the store like I had done a hundred times before, acknowledging the clerk as he rang me up for a packet of gum. This was the same guy I had seen day in and day out for the past six months. Average looking guy in his mid-20s. Pleasant enough.

I worked my way to the back of the store, stuck the bottle in the store microwave and pushed the "on" button. I stood there counting in my head, getting ready to pull the door open 15 or so seconds later. Just like I had many times before. Except this time, about 10 seconds in, I heard a loud pop. Not what I was expecting! I immediately pulled the microwave door open. To my horror, steaming hot urine was dripping off the top and sides of the microwave door. The bottle was now a hot, smoldering, stinky mess. What was left of it! The pressure in the bottle must have been too much. The bottle's entire contents covered every nook and cranny of the microwave. A quarter-inch pool of warm piss covered the turntable. *Did they turn up the power on the microwave? It has never done this before.*

I took one breath and gagged. The stench burned my eyes and my lungs at the same time. Like napalm. I pray I never have to smell something that toxic again. It quite literally smelled up the entire store within five seconds. I honestly felt like that store was done forever. Like they should have just taped it off with CAUTION – TOXIC WASTE tape, and condemned it unfit for habitation for the next 20 years. It smelled that bad.

I was thankful that the only person in the store was the poor clerk who no doubt had to clean up my mess. I walked out, head held low in shame, determined to never return to that store. The perfect footnote to the past three years of my life.

CHAPTER FIFTEEN

TIME TO GO

"I've said it too many times, and I still stand firm. You get what you put in, and people get what they deserve."

—Kid Rock (from 'Only God Knows Why')

I stood at the kitchen counter finely cutting up a white onion for the only dish I knew how to make. Spaghetti. Silence surrounded me. 8000 square feet of empty, lonely, rented misery. I had finally done it. I had finally managed to drive away the ones I loved the most.

It was the middle of the 2011 offseason, and my gorgeous wife was gone. The intoxicating laughter of my boys no longer radiated from the living room. The silence was killing me. I turned on sad 80s love songs. They rang out on the speakers throughout the house as I went about my "cooking." I felt baby tears stream down my face. No, it wasn't the onions. I was broken, alone, and depressed. My life had no purpose.

All the mistakes I had made since my first Adderall pill in Baltimore flooded my overwhelmed mind. I was sober. As a matter of fact, I had been completely sober since Baubi left with the boys a couple of weeks prior. And being sober made every past act that much clearer, further enhancing my misery. Knowing Baubi and the boys were in Houston with her family felt like a knife in my back. Yes, I deserved to be alone. But it still hurt deeply.

How can I possibly get my family back after doing the most unforgivable thing a husband and father can do? Up until two weeks earlier, my screw-ups seemed almost forgivable. In fact, I had convinced myself that I had never truly hurt anyone up until then. I had never put Baubi or my boys in danger. But that had all changed. Thinking back, I was disgusted at myself. *How could I have done such a stupid, selfish thing?*

The sun was setting through the dining room window as I sat down, plate of spaghetti in front of me. Before I could take the first bite, I heard the doorbell ring. *Who could this be at this hour? It's too late for any packages to be delivered,* I thought.

My heart skipped a beat. *It has to be Baubi and the kids!* I sprang out of the chair so fast that it fell backward, crashing on the hard tile floor behind me. I ran to the front door, fully expecting to see my beautiful family. I reached for the doorknob excitedly, and pulled the door open. I looked down for the baby blue eyes both boys inherit from me.

To my disappointment, standing where my family should have been was a woman wearing a flowered skirt, her arms completely hidden behind her back. I focused my gaze upward. Confused, I asked, "Can I help you?"

"Are you Aubrey Huff?" she asked.

"Yes ma'am, I am."

She pulled her hands from behind her as if she was about to pull a gun. I wish it had been. Instead, she thrust a large manila envelope toward me with an arrogant, evil smirk across her face. "You've been served," she said proudly.

I stood there for a moment, envelope in hand, then closed the door and turned slowly to face the long, darkened hallway. I felt like I had just been sucker-punched as I stumbled back toward the kitchen. The sad music sounded suicidal now as the reality of my situation was beginning to sink in. *I'm getting divorced. Following in the footsteps of my old man.* I had officially lost my family. And it was all my fault.

I remember that one of my biggest goals in life as an adolescent was to become a faithful, loving, and supportive husband to my future wife. I guess watching my mom go about it all alone all those years made me want to become someone who could make a difference in my wife's life. I wanted to become the husband that my father never was. I got sick to my stomach whenever I heard of men cheating on their wives, or worse still, leaving them. I instantly lost any respect I had for those men right then and there. In fact, as a kid, I had made a solemn vow to never, ever get divorced or cheat on my future wife.

That kid from long ago was now lost in a sea of emotional destruction. Chipped away at, like a cliff eroded by the constant motion of waves washing chunks off into the ocean. Now, I was just like any of the self-serving scumbags that I had resented so much growing up as a young man. I was no better than any of the men I had vowed to avoid becoming. And I couldn't blame anybody else.

Two weeks earlier.

We had moved into a gorgeous one-story, modern-style home just five minutes from Old Town Scottsdale, Arizona. That would be our home for the next six months. I was determined to get myself back into prime form there.

The 2011 season was in my rearview mirror now, and it was time to get my head and body in baseball shape again. I wanted to get back to my 2010 form where I was a man to be reckoned with on the field. A champion.

I was still using Adderall, but had backed the dosage off to my original 20 milligrams a day. I barely felt that low dosage now, but it was just enough to get me through my two-hour morning workouts. I was beginning to taper off my nightly beer drinking too, and was now starting to feel a bit more like the real me again. The offseason was going great. I began to engage with Jayce and Jagger in ways I never had before. Baubi and I, although still nowhere close to where we needed to be in our marriage, at least were on speaking terms again.

Any guy will tell you that it really doesn't take much for a guy to be happy. And I had all that I needed to put a smile back on my face. Things were looking up. I was beginning to really see improvements in my body, mind, and swing; I was confident I was on the right track. The rehab stint at Sundance seemed like a decade ago now.

Baubi walked through the front door in a noticeably sour mood one afternoon. I, of course, asked the absolute worst question any man could ask his wife. "What's wrong, honey, why the long face?"

The look she gave me could have burned through lead. "Why does anything have to be wrong just because I don't seem to be in a good mood?"

My response was something most men dare never say. "Oh, I get it. It must be that time of the month."

I wanted to eat those words the minute they spilled out of my mouth. Whatever was bothering her that day came out in pent-up rage that must have been building up for some time. She ripped into me, and I wasn't going to stand there and just take it. It was like World War III in our living room for what must have been 15 minutes. Right in front of the boys, too! Finally, Baubi looked at me with red, swollen eyes, and said in a trembling voice, "I need to get away from you for the day. I can trust you to handle the boys, can't I?"

With that, she stormed out the front door. The argument had my blood boiling, so I sat on the couch trying to let my blood pressure settle, watching the boys play Legos on the floor. They played with such joy and wonder. The look in their eyes gave off a sense of an inner peace and calmness that I desperately wanted in my life again. I climbed down off the couch to join them in some Lego building in hopes that some of their happiness would rub off on me. It didn't work. My simple mind craved more Adderall and maybe a few Bud Lights, too. I finally succumbed to my thoughts around four p.m. and I popped my second Adderall.

I was feeling the height of the high an hour and a half later. With a six-pack already down me, I microwaved some chicken nuggets for the boys. They watched *Caillou* on PBS Kids, and his obnoxious voice on the TV was really beginning to annoy the hell out of me. *What a whiny little turd,* I thought to myself as I brought Jayce, three, and Jagger, one, over to the dinner table. I didn't even fix anything for myself. My Bud Lights were filling me up quite nicely. I paced back and forth in the kitchen like a racehorse. Primed and ready to run, waiting for the gate to fling open.

I got the boys bathed. *I have to get out of this house!* I thought. I knew Baubi wouldn't be home until well after the kids were asleep. There was no getting out of the responsibility of getting them off to bed, which is no small chore for kids that age. I found myself getting angrier and angrier at my situation. I wanted no part of any responsibility in the state I was in. I wanted to party. To get out of the house. *Anywhere but here*, I thought to myself.

In my selfish state, I plopped the boys down on the couch around seven p.m. and began to look for a babysitter online. I found a company that looked reputable enough, although I didn't really bother reading the reviews, and called the first number I found. A friendly female voice answered, "Hello, how can I help you today?"

"Hi, my name is Aubrey, and I'm looking for a sitter for the night for my two boys, three and one. They will already be asleep when the sitter gets here, I just need someone here for safety's sake," I explained hurriedly.

"Well, sir, we have a number of different sitters in our registry. Would you like me to run through them for you?"

It took me less than a second to respond. "Absolutely not, just whoever can get here the fastest would be fine. I don't need a rundown. I'm sure she'll be fine."

"Um, okay, sir. I'll send someone over as fast as I possibly can. Thank you."

I hung up the phone, immediately grabbed the boys, and took them upstairs to their bedrooms. I got Jagger down first. He always fell asleep quickly and was out in just a few minutes. Jayce, on the other hand, loved to sit there and stare at the wall for a while as we snuggled. I should have been enjoying the intimacy of snuggling with my firstborn, but I sat there anxiously waiting for him to fall asleep so I could hit the town. All I could think of was the bar. The taste of that first cigarette. Maybe even a late night gentlemen's club. A place to clear my head and think.

I felt Jayce's dead weight on my shoulder. He was out. Just in time, too! The front doorbell rang.

The sitter looked innocent enough. Maybe a freshman in college. Short with brown hair, glasses, and a sweet little voice that would make anyone trust her. I quickly went over the situation with her.

"Thanks for getting here so quickly," I said. "My wife will be home soon and she will pay you. The boys are asleep in their bedrooms so you don't have to do anything. Watch TV; make yourself at home."

I found a blank sheet of paper from the desk and scribbled a note for Baubi:

Hey Babe,

Hope you had a fun day out without me. I know you needed it. I'm sorry I was such a prick today, but I promise I'll try to be better. Don't worry about the new babysitter when you walk in. I got her number from a teammate of mine. She is more than reputable. I did my home-work. Make sure you pay her. I needed to get out of the house as much as you did, believe me! Good night and I'll see you later.

Love you,
Aubrey

I taped the note to the door as I locked it behind me. My boys were fast asleep with a perfect stranger in the living room. I felt absolutely no remorse about my decision as I jumped into my car and drove into the night.

I have had many regrets in my life. This is the one single decision I regret the most. As a matter of fact, I feel my chest tighten and my palms sweat whenever I think of that poor choice.

When I look into Jayce and Jagger's eyes today, I'm filled with such love and compassion that it's hard for me to contain my emotions. Those two sweet boys have taught me how to love unconditionally. How to have a childlike faith. It was through my boys that I learned the value of selflessness. There is absolutely nothing on this Earth I wouldn't do for them. I thank God every day for blessing me with them. And I put them in harm's way that night. Back then I was Huffdaddy, my evil alter ego. Nobody was going to get in the way of me doing what I wanted to do. Not God. Not Baubi. And not the boys.

I stumbled back into the house around three a.m. and made my way upstairs. The boys were sleeping soundly. To my surprise, Baubi was sleeping next to Jagger, still fully clothed in the outfit I saw her in earlier. I was filled with a peace knowing they were all safe as I walked back down to the master bedroom and passed out.

I was awakened to the sound of kids crying and a *bump, bump, bump, bump* sound coming down the hallway toward the front door. I got out of bed and headed to the bathroom, not thinking too much about it. I stood there brushing my teeth, staring at myself in the mirror. *I look like hell.* My eyes were bloodshot and my hair was stale from no shower the night before. I reeked of beer and Marlboro Menthols.

Suddenly, my family appeared in the bathroom doorway behind me. I turned to greet them with a smile. The smile disappeared and my joy turned into panic as I locked eyes with Baubi. Baggy, sad, angry, red eyes. Two Tumi bags packed and ready to go. "Say good-bye to your father, boys."

I glanced down at their distraught faces. My heart sank. Jayce and Jagger walked slowly toward me. I slid down, my back against the bathroom sink, settling on the cold tile floor. I sat there, eye to eye with the boys. I grabbed them with both arms, pulling them in tight.

Jayce was first to speak. Through tears, he cried, "Daddy I'm going to miss you." Tears streamed down my face and his. I looked up to Baubi, the boys still in my grasp. Her expression remained frozen in resolute disgust as I pleaded with her. "Please, honey, don't do this!"

"I'm sorry but you have given me no choice; you have put our kids in danger. You've made my life miserable for long enough. There's no way you're going to endanger my children. We're leaving." She paused for a moment. "Let's go, boys. Time to go."

I watched them vanish out the bathroom toward the front door. I sat there in disbelief. *This can't be happening. This has to be a dream.* The front door slammed, snapping me out of it. This was real. And it was gut-wrenching.

I sat on that cold floor in just my boxers for what seemed like hours, crying uncontrollably. I hope and pray my friends, that you never have to endure that feeling. Watching the ones you love the most walk out. The emptiness. I had never ever felt that kind of pain. I remember thinking to myself, *If this is hell then I'd better get used to it.*

Two weeks later I was served.

It took me a solid couple of days to get it together. I had to get clean, and I knew it. I made a promise to myself right there and then to get clean and get them back. And I was well on my way until that knock at the door.

Now, with my family gone, I had nothing to live for. Starting back up on Adderall was an easy choice. I needed something to occupy my guilty, depressed mind, and the little orange-and-white pills were the only thing that could take the pain away, if only for a little while.

Baseball was the very last thing on my mind as I began the process of finding a divorce attorney. I was sure to lose millions, but in all honesty, I couldn't have cared less. *She can have it all,* I thought. *I deserve it.* I deserved to be broke, poor, and alone. I grew up as a young boy in a trailer park in Texas, so I figured *What the hell, I'll go back to one.*

I stood around for a few days. Feeling sorry for myself. Desperately trying to drown my sorrows. The days dragged. I got tired of that routine pretty quickly. *I have to get back in shape. Get my career back on track,* I thought.

With my family in Houston, I began training hard for the season while doubling up on my dose during the day. With that dosage, the monster inside me had no choice but to come out. I was uncontrollable that entire month of January. Nobody was home to answer to. No responsibility and no shame. I would work out for two or three hours each morning. Some nights I would go out by myself to a club or gentleman's club to kill the boredom. Most nights I found myself playing blackjack at the Talking Stick Casino in Scottsdale.

It was a random Wednesday night February 8th, six days before Valentine's Day, and just two weeks before spring training camp. I found myself at two a.m. at the casino. I had taken out 10 grand from the ATM to play blackjack. I was up 27 thousand dollars in no time flat. And I lost it all just as fast as I had won it, including my original 10 grand.

I walked out of that casino toward my car, high, dejected, and drunk. I had no business hopping into my car that night, but in the state I was in, I didn't care. I wouldn't have even minded if I hit a tree killing myself on the way home, just as long as I didn't kill someone else.

I was just a few blocks away from home when I saw a flash of red and blue in my rearview mirror. Panic rushed through my body. I pulled over to the side of the road, convinced I would be spending the night in jail.

The officer approached my car, and I rolled down my window. "Sir, can you step out of the vehicle, please?" he asked calmly. The adrenaline sobered me up instantly as I stood next to my car door. He continued, "You been drinking tonight, sir?"

I contemplated saying no, but knew he would no doubt know I was lying, so I said, "Yes, sir, I had a few at the casino and lost 10 grand fairly quickly, so decided to call it a night." I maintained eye contact with him confidently the entire time as if I had nothing to hide. He stood there, peering deep into my soul, as if in a staring contest.

Finally, in a soft voice, he said, "Okay, Aubrey, just be more careful next time. You completely ran a stop sign back there, you know? By the way, good luck this season. I'm a huge Giants fan."

He walked away. I sat back behind the wheel and breathed a huge sigh of relief.

Something has to change. This is getting ridiculous, I thought. I was spiraling out of control.

That night as I stumbled toward my bed, I felt this sickening presence surround my soul. It was a feeling of hopelessness and of darkness. My mind began to race with the feeling that someone was watching me. Someone...something evil. My soul was overcome with worthlessness.

I fell to my knees at the edge of my bed and began to cry uncontrollably at the top of my voice. In my despair, somewhere in the back of my mind and from the depths of my heart, I felt the need to pray to God. I hadn't spoken to him since rehab a year prior.

With hands clenched together, and eyes closed tightly, still swollen and soaked with tears, I prayed like I had never prayed before, with passion and sincerity, "Lord, I have nothing left. No family, no happiness, no love, no future. I hate the man I have become."

I instantly began to feel an inner peace as I continued. "Please Lord, forgive me for all the sins I've committed, and all the damage I've done to my friends, and especially my family. Lord, I pray by your grace and mercy that you can give them back to me, and change me into the man I know you want me to be. I know it's asking a lot, but Lord, I know you can work miracles. Lord, I can't kick these pills by myself. I've tried rehab. I've tried cold turkey. I just can't do it. I need you to help me kick this addiction."

I sobbed. Tears dripping down my arms, soaking the mattress near my elbows.

"Please Lord, I beg you! I'm going to prove to you my obedience." I got up and walked into the bathroom. I grabbed my pill bottle and headed toward the toilet. I emptied the bottle into the bowl and watched the little pills sink to the bottom. I flushed with zero hesitation and watched the little eddy current swirl them around, washing them down the s-bend.

"Lord, I know by your love, mercy, grace, and forgiveness, I will be healed. I pray that I'll never have the desire to take another Adderall as long as I live. It's in your holy name I pray, Lord Jesus. Amen."

I walked back toward my bed. I felt absolutely amazing. Like a 200-pound weight had just been lifted off my shoulders. I sank into the soft mattress and slept like a baby.

Thursday, February 9th, 2012. The next day.

I awoke surprisingly not hungover and in a fantastic mood. Adderall didn't even cross my mind until later in the evening.

It was then that I realized I had gone the entire day without wanting a pill.

I knew I had prayed the night before for God to end my addiction, but *no way he could have healed me so quickly,* I reasoned. The next day, same thing. No desire for a pill. And the next day.

How could this be? Could Jesus really have cured me overnight? I racked my brain, trying to think of an answer. There was no other explanation I could come up with. Jesus must have heard my prayer. And he must have answered! I was all in.

I began reading the Bible even though I understood barely any of it. And I began praying daily for God to turn me into the man he wanted me to become. I prayed diligently every day for him to soften Baubi's heart, and for her to forgive me. I prayed he would help me become a loving, attentive husband and father. And I prayed for him to return my family to me, if that was his will.

I did not feel like I deserved any of what I was praying for. But I had nowhere else to turn. And no one else to put my faith in.

The Aubrey Huff from just before college returned just days before the start of spring training. I was extremely nervous to play naked. I was on my knees daily, praying for courage and strength. A little voice in my head taunted me, and feelings of insecurity crept in. *We can't miss the playoffs again this year.* The old me was shy, soft, and unconfident. Not exactly the traits you needed to carry into a Major League Baseball season. But that would be the exact Aubrey Huff who would go into battle that 2012 season.

Walking into the Giants clubhouse in Arizona for the first day of camp felt all too familiar. Just like the year before, I was committed to stay clean. This time felt different though. Yes, I was determined to never use Adderall again. And yes, I was convinced I would get my family back. But this time, I felt absolutely sure I would succeed. I had God on my side.

CHAPTER SIXTEEN
MISERY OF A CHAMPION

"All it takes is a beautiful fake smile to hide an injured soul and they will never notice how broken you really are."

—Robin Williams

The first chapter ended with me touching down in Tampa after a brutal, three-hour red-eye flight home from New York. It was April 22nd, 2012, and I had fled New York, abandoning my teammates, convinced I was knocking on death's door.

Guilt got the better of me while I waited at the baggage claim. I felt compelled to call Bruce Bochy to explain my absence. I told him I had a family emergency and had to leave town, but that I would be back to meet the team for the next series against the Reds in Cincinnati, Ohio. He completely understood and wished me well. "Hope everything's okay," he said before we hung up.

I was breathing a little easier now the wave of panic had passed. I wasn't sure what had happened. I just figured that perhaps it was something I had eaten, or maybe someone had slipped something in my drink the night before. All I knew was that I felt so much better now and was excited to see my family and finally relax in my own home for one full day.

I had not called Baubi to give her a heads-up, figuring that a phone call in my state would have been a bad idea. We had been chatting on the phone more and more trying to figure out how to make the separation work. She was praying day and night and felt that God was telling her to not give up on our marriage, even when everything, and everyone, was telling her "No way!" I was praying constantly too. My prayers were being answered as God was slowly softening her heart towards me, helping her see my strong, kind heart underneath all the lies and deception.

Baubi hated me. She had every right to never trust me again. In fact I was convinced she could never forgive me or get over all the pain I had caused her over the years. She had grown up with a father that suffered from bipolar disorder. He was never there for her. Some of the most vivid memories Baubi had of her father were of him violently unleashing his frustrations on her older brother Charles. As he grew more distant and withdrew deeper into himself, her mother had to step up to the plate to become the sole provider. Like me, Baubi essentially grew up without a father, and now she must have felt like she had married someone just like him, a selfish prick living inside his head, preoccupied with everything *but* his family. As much as it pained her, she knew she couldn't let her boys experience the same pain she felt growing up without a father. She would have been long gone if the boys were not in the picture. Her heart was telling her to give us one last shot. The divorce was still in the works and she figured that if I continued to be a douchebag, she would simply let the process continue.

Even though her family and friends were calling her nuts considering taking me back, she felt it was a risk worth taking for her boys. They were convinced I could never change and that I would just keep on breaking her heart over and over again. Who could blame them? Baubi's mother Naomi was the only one who respected and approved of her decision, despite all she had personally suffered at the hands of her nonexistent husband.

Baubi knew that there was no way we could make our marriage work while living on opposite sides of the country. She had finally made the decision earlier that month to reunite our little family in San Francisco. In fact, she was halfway through packing for the move to the west coast when I showed up unannounced and in a state of panic that morning. Needless to say, she was shocked to see me.

My children were excited, but as much as I wanted to spend time and play with them, all I could do was sleep the whole day away. I lay on the bed, drowsy, eyes heavy. Baubi sat on the edge of the bed, a concerned look on her face. I briefly clued her in on what had happened. She told me in no uncertain terms that I needed to clean up my act. Even though I was Adderall-free now, I was still numbing myself with alcohol daily. She was convinced I had suffered a panic attack and I didn't have the strength to disagree. I nodded, chalked it up as a one-time thing, and drifted off.

I was feeling pretty good the next day. I felt rested and excited to get back at it as I lined up my flight to Cincinnati for the following morning.

I woke up around eight a.m., ate a quick breakfast and got myself mentally prepared to reunite with my team. I heard the hum of the Town Car as it pulled into the driveway just as I zipped up my last bag. The sound of that zipper closing must have triggered something because suddenly, the same feelings I had experienced in New York returned. My heart began to race, my mind lost control, panic began to set in once again.

Here we go again, I thought. *There is no way you are gonna get me on that plane.* I honestly told myself right then and there that if I was to quit baseball forever and lose my contract, I wouldn't care. All I wanted was to feel normal again.

I shuffled out the front door, slipped the driver a hundred for his trouble, and sent him away. My panic disappeared down our street with him. I put two and two together. *Baseball is what is bringing these attacks on.* I called my trainers in San Francisco and laid out the scene in as much detail as I could recall. They immediately had me check in with a local therapist in Tampa. I remember sitting in that cold air-conditioned room anxiously waiting for answers. The prognosis? Severe anxiety disorder. The treatment: 20 milligrams of Xanax a day.

In my mind, people who had panic attacks were mentally weak people who couldn't cope with life. I never thought of myself as a mentally weak person. As a matter of fact, if anything, I thought I overflowed with confidence, a man's type of man, the life of the party. The guy known for keeping it loose in the clubhouse. I never thought in my wildest dreams that I would be taking Xanax for panic attacks. But underneath the confident and relaxed surface, a violent storm of insecurity, fear, doubt, and worry must have been brewing for years.

I missed the three-game series in Cincinnati and it took two Xanax and my family in tow to finally get me on that plane to San Francisco for the beginning of the home stand against the Padres.

When I rejoined the team a few days later, I was a ghost. I had gone from a 2010 leader on a World Series–winning team to a cautionary tale almost overnight. I was placed on the 60-day disabled list for anxiety, becoming a bench player who had lost his job to young Brandon Belt. And that was fine by me! I didn't want to play anymore. I was done!

I felt like a zombie with the Xanax pumping through my system that entire year. After I completed my DL stint and returned to the team, things just got worse. Pitcher Matt Cain threw a perfect game against the Houston Astros at home in San Francisco on June 13th. As the final out was made, the entire bench rushed the field, and I, being the athlete I am, couldn't quite make it over the railing that protected the dugout. My left foot got caught in the rail netting and I fell four feet, landing with my full weight on my right kneecap. Agonizing pain shot through my whole leg. Trying to stand up just made it worse.

I had to crawl to the bathroom the next morning, being careful not to bend or put pressure on my knee. Turned out I had a deep bone bruise that put me on crutches for a couple of weeks, and sent me back to the minors for rehab. I had a feeling the Giants weren't exactly in any hurry to get me back.

I finally made it back to the big leagues just as the Giants were in hot pursuit of another playoff drive. The guys worked their asses off to clench the division title that year. I had done nothing to help them and did not feel I deserved to be on the playoff roster. I was fully expecting to be left off, and to be completely honest, I was secretly hoping not to make it because I knew that the pressure and intensity of the playoffs were sure to heighten my already-growing anxiety. Bruce added me on out of pity.

It had been a few days since I took a Xanax, but I carried one with me in a little plastic bag in the back of my baseball pants pocket, just in case I felt an attack coming on. I didn't want to risk wasting precious minutes, walking back to the locker room to get my hands on it if I needed it.

Bottom of the 8th inning. Game one. 2012 World Series at home in San Francisco against the Detroit Tigers. Brandon Crawford had just lined out to center field for out number two.

We were up 8-1. We clearly had this game under control. No one on base. Perfect time for Bruce to put me in. We had nothing to lose. "Huffy. You're hitting for Timmy." he barked. I sprang out of my seat and made my way from half way down the bench to the end of the dugout, reaching for my helmet and hurriedly strapping on my batting gloves. I hustled up to the on-deck circle and took a few quick swings in an attempt to get loose.

Rick Porcello stood there eyeing me from the mound, like a gator eyeing a chicken. Rick was an awesome guy. He was very laid back, especially for his young age. I enjoyed hanging out with him the most during my brief time in Detroit. I didn't stand a chance against him. I was a mental midget.

First pitch. His trademark heavy sinker. I swung and made contact weakly off the end of the bat. The ball sputtered towards third base. A ground out. I shuffled back to the dugout, head held low, staring at the green grass in shame. *There is no way Bruce is going to let me bat again* I thought. I had this sinking feeling as I crossed in front of the pitcher's mound that I had just had my last major league at bat. I glanced up at the crowd and soaked it all in. The smells, sights and sounds of the stadium. The atmosphere. I glanced at my teammates, all lined up on the dugout railing as they looked upon me with pity. Embarrassed for me. They had all witnessed my train wreck since the panic attack firsthand, and they knew, like I did, it was all over for Aubrey Huff.

Bruce seemed genuinely happy when he first told me I had made the playoff roster. He was excited for me. I am sure he knew in his heart I was done playing baseball. He wanted to give me one last hurrah. The simple fact he took me into consideration tells you everything you need to know about the kind of stand-up guy he is, and also explains the amazing success the Giants have experienced under his leadership.

The rest of the team was on top of their game. They were all so amped to be in the World Series. For me, the adrenaline, the excitement, everything that I had experienced just two years before was gone. I felt like an outcast.

Game three was well-pitched between Ryan Vogelsong and Anibal Sanchez. We came out victorious, beating them 2-0, putting us up three games to none. The Tigers had waited since 1984 to lift a World Series trophy and now they needed to win out. We had this in the bag and were closing in on a second championship win in three years.

Bruce could tell I was feeling down on myself. He came up to me after the game and said "Huffy, I am not sure, but I am thinking about starting you at DH tomorrow. So get to the field ready." I was stoked. A chance to play in a clinching game. *Maybe I can end my career on something other than a feeble ground out.* I hardly slept that night.

October 28th, 2012. Game four. I felt the nervous excitement coursing through my veins on the bumpy bus ride to Comerica Park that morning. *Wow. Another World Series.* I loved to DH. I already wrote about that. And now, I would get the chance to be a hero and go out on top. My phone buzzed in my back pocket rudely interrupting my thoughts of glory. It was a text message from Bruce. "Sorry Huffy. I decided to DH Ryan Theriot instead today." Talk about a kick in the nuts!

Déjà vu crept into my mind. This felt very familiar. The only other time I had had the rug pulled out from under me like that was also in Detroit. I don't blame Bruce for making that decision now, but in the heat of the moment, I was frustrated and disappointed. I didn't understand why he would use a right handed batter to DH against a right handed pitcher.

It was a chilly night in Detroit. I snuggled up on the bench watching the guys take the field in front of a crazed home crowd. I couldn't help but see the passion that Hunter Pence had. That sparkling look of determination and excitement in his eyes. The bounce in his step in the dugout right before he took the field for the big game. I could tell he really loved the game. I glanced over toward the edge of the dugout and eyed Buster Posey sitting next to Madison Bumgarner. They were now the team stars with big, bright futures ahead of them. I was so jealous of the charisma, leadership, and passion they exuded. Me? I was now the salty washed-up veteran at the end of his career.

Top of the 10th. My replacement Ryan Theriot led off with a single to right off Phil Coke. He would prove to be the winning run when Marco Scutaro's single scored him from second base putting us ahead 4-3. Bochy had made the right call. Theriot took the field with a fire in his eyes. He made all the difference that day.

Bottom of the tenth, two outs. The 2012 Triple Crown–winning Miguel Cabrera strolled to the plate. *One swing from his mighty bat could tie this thing up.* The dugout sat on pins and needles, anxiously waiting for the final out to charge the field to celebrate. My face was sore now from all the fake smiles and laughs. I wanted the whole thing to be over and done with so I could begin my new life. A life without baseball and all the anxiety it brought with it. Sergio Romo threw a 3-2 fastball right down the middle, freezing Miguel. That pitch crowned us 2012 World Series champs.

The dugout and every Giants player on the field charged the mound to celebrate, much to the disdain of the silenced Tigers crowd. I was last to reach the pile, looking around for someone to hug. But I stood there like the last kid picked at kickball. Nobody even knew I was there as I watched from a distance. Many of my teammates had just won their first World Series. I knew what that felt like and I tried to be happy for them. But try as I might, I just couldn't. The Xanax was pushing me down into an emotionless abyss.

I didn't want to celebrate. I was ashamed to be there, embarrassed even. I was faking every moment, and as I walked off the field at Tiger Stadium that night I knew without a doubt that it would be the last time I would ever set foot on a Major League Baseball field. The entire team celebrated in the clubhouse, spraying champagne. Everyone except me. I didn't feel I deserved to. I was first to leave the clubhouse. And I didn't hang out with the team that night for the post-game party.

The season was over. The World Series was over. And so was my career. I could finally breathe, the source of my anxiety gone for good. Or so I thought.

Many people tell me today, "Man, Aubrey, it must have been awesome going out a World Series champ." All I can say is, "Yep. Sure was." But in reality, that was one of the most difficult moments of my life.

Funny what a difference just two years can make. After winning our first World Series title in 2010, I had proudly waved my red rally thong in front of a million-plus adoring fans during our championship parade. I was a fun-loving teammate and a true leader. Now, at the 2012 parade I was embarrassed to even be there. I have a picture in my storage closet that perfectly illustrates my state during that celebration. The entire team is gathered exuberantly around the World Series trophy on stage in front of a sea of orange and black. I am standing in the background, slightly out of focus, with my eyes looking down and a frown that I couldn't control.

I wanted to be happy, just like all the fans, teammates, coaches, and staff. But I couldn't. A belly full of Xanax took away my anxiety, but it also suppressed every other emotion, making it literally impossible to feel any joy. Still, being a zombie sounded far better than another panic attack.

I knew the Giants would not pick up my $10-million team option for the following season. We were renting a home for the offseason, and were driving there when my phone rang. It was assistant general manager Bobby Evans confirming what I already knew. Relief came instantly. The weight of the world lifted off my shoulders as I drove through that lonely desert with my family, knowing that I had my entire life ahead of me. I could do whatever I wanted now. It was a freeing moment, and I felt a sense of excitement for the first time in a long time. I had no idea what I wanted to do with the rest of my life, all I knew was that it was going to have nothing to do with baseball.

Ask any ex-professional athlete and they will tell you that transitioning into real life is hard. I lived in a fairy tale world for so long with everyone catering to my every need that leaving the game for the real world felt weird. Like my identity was stripped from me. And with it, my manhood.

My transition seemed to be going well until 2013 spring training started. I hadn't missed one in 15 years, and now I was beginning to feel on edge about what my future held. True, I was free to do whatever I wanted, but I desperately wanted to achieve more. Baseball had been my Plan A my whole life. I was simply not equipped to dive into another career. In my growing anxiety, I began to drink. Again. The alcohol mixed with Xanax seemed to curb my anxiety, but depression was really starting to sink in now. And I was so confused. Here I was retired at 36, having achieved everything I had ever wanted and then some. *Why can't I just be content and happy?*

I just didn't understand it. *What did I do wrong, God? You delivered me from my Adderall addiction. You gave me my family back. Why am I still so depressed? Why do I feel so empty?*

I had to find a new passion in life. A new dream to grind at. Another goal to achieve. So I started throwing all kinds of different lines in the water. I worked at 95.7 *The Game,* a sports talk radio show in San Francisco. That lasted four short months. I found that line of work too critical and negative in nature for my liking. As a matter of fact, I grew to hate it so much that I was having panic attacks daily because of the discontent it added to my life at home. I tried volunteering at a local high school to see if I would enjoy the coaching side of baseball. I hated it too. I literally wanted nothing to do with baseball anymore. I even took a stab at network marketing for about a year, but I just couldn't get passionate about it.

I was at my wits' end. I had spent my whole career sure of my identity. Now I had none. I was no longer Aubrey Huff, the pro baseball player. I had enjoyed the certainty of a schedule, knowing where I had to be each day. Now I woke up each morning not even sure what I should do that next hour. I had lived my life as a man on a mission. Now that mission was gone. I can only imagine what those serving our country must feel like when they come back and try to get back to a "normal" civilian life.

No matter what I tried, I knew I could never reproduce the passion and excitement that baseball created. And I knew I could never replace the adrenaline rush 40,000 people in the stands screaming my name brought.

I began suffering massive panic attacks daily, except this time I couldn't blame baseball. I was panicked about my future during the day, and dragged under by mind-bending depression at night. I had never been so low in my life and felt like God was just as far away from me as he had ever been. I even began to entertain using Adderall again.

I had finally reached a tipping point. Life didn't seem worth it anymore! You no doubt have heard about pro athletes that couldn't adjust to the hell that is the real world, tragically taking their own lives. I was beginning to think this was the only way out for me as well.

I saw no future for me. I had a smart, loving, supportive, forgiving, gorgeous wife and two handsome, happy boys who loved their dad with all their hearts. But something in my head told me they deserved better.

Let me paint the picture for you. Late October 2014. Another gorgeous day in sunny San Diego, one straight out of the visitors and convention bureau's brochure. It might as well have been cloudy and miserable because that summed up my mood better. I stood next to Baubi at the kitchen counter as she labored, a beautiful smile on her face, cooking a healthy dinner for her three boys. I felt a knot in my stomach. A wave of cold sweat, then a hot flush washed over me. My heart began to race, and my breathing became labored. *Great! Another panic attack.* Jayce and Jagger played happily on the living room floor, oblivious. Life couldn't have been more perfect, but my mind only saw misery. I felt the blood drain from my head and the color leave my face. I had to retreat from the kitchen. *I can't let my family see me like this again.*

I stepped into the bedroom closet, closing the door behind me. I had had enough. I didn't even want to take my Xanax.

I wanted to feel the misery, to own it. I stood there for a few minutes, palms sweating, each arm feeling like it weighed a hundred pounds as it dangled by my side. I punched the code into my safe and grabbed my .357 Magnum. The soft beige carpet felt like a pillow as I dropped to my knees, staring at myself in the full-length mirror on the closet wall, tears rolling down my face. The panic attack was peaking.

I cradled the gun in the palm of my hands and studied the engraving on the cold stainless steel barrel as it reflected the cold lighting in the closet: Smith & Wesson, Made in USA. Springfield, Mass.

I looked up at myself in the mirror again. The man who looked back at me with sullen eyes seemed like a scared little boy desperate to look like a real man, complete with a buzz cut, rough goatee, tattoos that ran down both arms, and a tight wifebeater. I was so tired of the fight in my head. Sick of the panic attacks I was suffering daily now. And I couldn't handle the depression that came each evening as the sun set. I was tired of life!

The gun felt heavy in my hand, especially with six hollow point Critical Defense 125 grain rounds in the revolver. I balanced it carefully in my right hand as I pulled the hammer back.

My knees were burning now as the carpet fibers dug into my kneecaps. *I'm so tired of the constant worrying.* I didn't understand why I worried. *What the hell do I have to worry about? I have everything my heart has ever desired.* I entertained the thought of blowing my brains out for a second. I wasn't at the point where I was going to do it quite yet, but I wasn't too far away. I simply wanted to practice the steps leading up to it, if you will.

I brought the fully loaded Magnum up to my temple and stared at myself dead in the eyes in the mirror. They were bloodshot red and filled with tears. *Just a simple squeeze of the trigger to end it all.*

The pain, anxiety, and misery would finally be gone. I thought of Baubi. I thought of the kids. They would be set for life and would not have to worry about money. *But am I being selfish even thinking about leaving them like this?* I visualized my wife and kids finding me in the closet, brain fragments and blood everywhere. Their father lying there on the floor without a head. Then I thought about the pain I had felt as a little kid, heck, the pain I *still* felt thirty years after losing my father. *Do I really want my boys to feel that pain?* I wrestled with my mind. A voice in my left ear urged me to do it, *"You don't have a future, Aubrey. Just pull the trigger. You won't feel a thing!"* A voice in my right ear whispered gently, *"Don't do it Aubrey, your life is just beginning, you have so much to live for."* I glanced away from the sorry sight in the mirror and saw the twenty-plus custom-made suits for road trips hanging neatly in a row, a reminder of my playing days. I literally had everything that 99.9 percent of the men in the world would die for. And I was almost willing to blow it all away.

A sudden thought hijacked my mind. *My dad was murdered with a .357 Magnum.*

CHAPTER SEVENTEEN
GET BUSY...

"Consider it pure joy, my brothers and sisters, whenever you face trials of many kinds, because you know that the testing of your faith produces perseverance. Let perseverance finish its work so that you may be mature and complete, not lacking anything."

— James 1: 2-4 (NIV)

I jerked the gun away from my temple violently, as if I had just woken up from a bad dream. I eased the hammer back, locked the safety, and set it down carefully. Seeing it sink into the carpet near my knees suddenly made me angry. I mean I got really pissed. I hissed, "God, why are you putting me through this?" I thought, *If this is how you treat your followers, Lord, then screw this!* There had to be no God if I was feeling that way.

I prayed, if you could call it that. I felt the cold concrete push back at my knees through the carpet. *I'm already on my knees,* I thought. *I may as well see what he has to say about my situation.* As my anger overtook me, my prayer was more like that of a rebellious teenager spitting venom at his father. I screamed at God at the top of my lungs, tears of misery flowing, blurring my vision.

"Why God? Why the hell are you doing this to me? When are you going to relieve me of this misery?" Every joint in my body ached. My head was throbbing. I felt depleted and completely defeated. "I thought when I asked you into my heart all this was supposed to go away!" I was sad, confused, scared, and mad.

I lay on my back and took in a lungful of air. I allowed myself to breathe again. I was still sobbing, but I felt my heartbeat slow as I began to calm down. The anxiety lifted and my tears slowly dried on my warm face. I lay there motionless staring up at the ceiling. The bright light stung my eyes. I wanted to get up and turn the lights out so I could sit quietly in cool darkness, but I couldn't risk it. My body was finally calm. *I can't budge. What if the panic comes back?* The silence in that closet was eerie. I could hear my heart pulsating, the blood rushing through my veins with every squeeze.

I asked God again, calmly this time, "Lord, why am I feeling like this? Why am I entertaining killing myself? Please, Lord. I desperately need an answer. Is this all part of your master plan? If it is, I sure as hell don't get it!"

The silence was deafening. A thought came rushing into my mind from out of nowhere. It was unmistakable. *"Aubrey, if you want my perfect peace, you have to give up control and have faith in me."*

My friends, when I asked Christ into my life in February 2012, my Adderall addiction disappeared immediately. But what followed was easily the worst baseball season of my life. My last.

If I knew about the 60 documented side effects of Adderall before popping my first pill in Baltimore so many years before, I never would have done it. I certainly didn't know the science behind it then, but I now know that Adderall was exactly what started my panic attacks in the first place.

The generic name for Adderall is amphetamine / dextroamphetamine. Speed. According to the maker of Adderall, Teva Pharmaceuticals, one common side effect is anxiety! Reading the complete list of side effects would be entertaining if I did not know firsthand how serious many of them are. I won't bore you with details, but they include: seeing, hearing, or feeling things that are not there, sudden loss of consciousness, sweating, tightness in the chest, trouble breathing, nausea, dizziness, and double vision.

I had felt like absolute hell each morning in the midst of my addiction as the dose from the day before wore off. Popping another pill was the only way to fix it. It was not until I got off Adderall, and detoxed it out of my system that I was able to feel the full weight of its side effects. With nothing to mask them, all the symptoms of a panic attack were now free to wage war on my mind and body. Supposedly, increasing the dosage means never having to face these symptoms head-on, but how much speed could my body handle before self-destructing? Left unchecked, and under different circumstances, I am convinced I would have eventually either blown an artery, or my brains out.

Sure, God took away my addiction in 2012, but here I was a new Christian, an unrepentant alcoholic and drug addict, going through one of the worst years of my life, regretting my decision to even accept Jesus into my heart in the first place. I honestly believed that my life was better without Jesus. I certainly *felt* better without him!

That thought bugged me for a long time and it's only recently I realized that I was living a lie that whole time. I was a Christian Atheist. Although I believed God was up there, I certainly wasn't living my life like it. I had never truly surrendered, and was still trying to control everything, praying only when I was sad, needing a miracle, or when things didn't go my way. I certainly never prayed for others. I was a fake, self-absorbed, hypocrite Christian, the kind that turns people off Christianity.

When I was in the thick of my anxiety and depression, I met with a psychiatrist in San Diego once a week. After about 10 sessions at 275 bucks a pop I asked, "Hey Doc, have you ever had anxiety or depression?" He gave me an odd look. "No, Aubrey. But I've had a lot of schooling on the subject." I pressed him further, "Doc do you believe in God?" He looked confused, "Well no Aubrey I don't. Why do you ask?" "Well, I believe that God is allowing me to go through this to turn me into the man he wants me to be, and that I will be freed from this pain in his good timing." I responded confidently. The look he gave me was one of doubt and cynicism. "Aubrey, I'm sorry but I just don't believe that there is a God up there that can help you. You have to be able to help yourself...to find the root cause of what is causing these attacks so that you can rid yourself of this." That would be the last time we ever saw each other.

I realized I was wasting my time, and money! The degrees hanging on the wall in his office were pretty impressive, and I am sure he meant well, but I knew that beyond prescribing medication, he had zero clue how to really help me. And I certainly knew that his discrediting my beliefs wasn't going to make me better anytime soon.

I know from experience that you can't learn to hit a baseball by reading a book or listening to a coach talking about it. And you definitely can't help someone that suffers from depression or anxiety unless you have been through the trenches yourself and found a way to crawl out alive.

My family and friends were no better, even though they truly cared for me and were concerned for my wellbeing. They wanted to help, but like my therapist, they could not relate to what I was going through. I remember lying in bed staring at the ceiling in a catatonic depressed state one afternoon. I didn't hear Baubi walk in. She stood at the edge of the bed, clearly frustrated, barking at me, "Wow babe! You've got to get out of your head! Look around you, you have a great life. There are people out there dying of cancer! You don't have it *that* bad. Get off your butt and do something!" I knew she was right. She made it sound so easy, but my legs felt like they weighed 200 pounds each. I felt like I couldn't crawl out of bed even if I wanted to! I knew she meant well, but her attempt to help just angered me and made me feel even more depressed. *She just doesn't get it,* I reasoned. Fact is, most people never will.

So many people ask me after I speak about my journey, "Aubrey your story has inspired me so much. I suffer too, like you have. Please tell me. How did you do it? How did you turn it all around?"

I was now fumbling through life without a routine or plan of any kind, and as I emerged from my closet on that dark suicidal day, I knew that had to change. I desperately needed a plan now.

I marched straight into my office, scrounged around for a blank piece of paper and a number two pencil, and outlined what would become my new normal. I committed to the new plan no matter how difficult it became or how long it took. Weeks, months, years even. Yeah, as you might have guessed, it took years!

I have refined that plan, but the essentials remain the same today. You may not believe what I believe or agree with everything in here, and if you are struggling from anxiety or depression, or are having suicidal thoughts, please get help right away. I just know that these steps are what helped me make it out of the trenches alive, and I still follow them each day as best I can. I knew back then that there is no magic bullet for dealing with real pain, and that just like baseball, it was going to take a lot of hard work and discipline. But I was ready for the challenge.

"Aubrey, if you want my perfect peace, you have to give up control and have faith in me." *What the hell does that mean? Give up control?* I loved the sound of 'perfect peace.' In fact, I was desperate for it, but giving up control is painful for me. I don't even let anyone else drive. I want to be the one with my hands on the wheel. I had absolutely no idea *how* to give up control. I needed help. So I decided right then I would wake up early every day, hand the wheel over to God, and ask for his help. Pray.

Now, I am not trying to cram my beliefs down your throat, but even today, I pray the minute I wake up, thanking God for another day of life. I grab a coffee and sit with my bible until a verse resonates with me. I write that passage down and meditate on it all day, looking for ways to apply it.

The Bible may as well have been written in Greek when I first started, but I couldn't go backwards. I had to be faithful, and give this God thing a real chance. Eventually, it made more sense, and now I really look forward to the peace it brings me most mornings. The rest of my days were pretty mundane–like I mentioned in the beginning of the book, I was basically a househusband, a far cry from the big leagues. But these verses made my days more tolerable.

I have had so many people tell me I needed to read the Bible throughout my life. I thought they were all whack jobs at the time. I remember one particular teammate back in the minor leagues, in AA Orlando. He sat next to me on the ten-hour bumpy bus ride from Orlando to Knoxville. I felt like hell from the night before and smelled even worse as he beat me over the head relentlessly with bible verses, showing me the evil of my ways. If his plan was to draw me closer to God, it backfired. I felt even worse about myself and was fully convinced I was going to burn in hell. I see now he had a point, but his approach sucked. Let me just say that if you bump into me at a coffee shop in San Diego, don't worry, I'm a lot of things, but I am not a hypocrite. I won't be throwing any bible verses at you, especially knowing how truly selfish I had been much of my life, thinking only about how I was feeling, how I was doing, and what I was going to do with my future.

I took Jayce and Jagger to a game here in San Diego not long ago. I was lucky to have a chance to walk them into the Giants's dugout so they could meet some of my ex-teammates. It was fun to see the looks of admiration on their faces. As we got ready to say "bye" to the team, Buster Posey, easily one of the nicest and most talented guys I had ever had the pleasure to be teammates with, looked me square in the eyes, and with a dead serious tone said, "Huffy. What happened to you? You're so nice now!" That really struck a chord with me. I couldn't help but think to myself, *I must have seemed like the biggest horse's ass to him when we played together.*

I had spent my life going to great lengths to shield the pain and torment in my mind by building a wall of sarcasm around me. It was my way of making sure no one got even close to knowing the real me. On paper, throughout my career, I appeared to be one of the best players on most teams I played for. But deep down inside, I was terrified of true leadership and responsibility, and would have probably dropped dead of a heart attack if I were ever asked to be team captain. Being the team jester ensured that would never happen. I had dropped that act now, and Buster noticed. But it wasn't easy.

I believe that sarcasm is negativity's little brother, and if indulged in too much, will lead you down a negative wormhole. My sarcasm on and off the field grew into a serious cloud of negativity that followed me into my retirement. My mind would be fully convinced Baubi was going to be raped and killed and my kids kidnapped, whenever they left the house. My bleak view of life was dragging me down. It had to stop.

As cliché as it sounds, I had to start rewiring my brain for positivity. I stopped watching television and started reading inspirational books and listening to motivational speakers instead.

Javier Lopez, an ex-fellow-Giant, would always wear a rubber band on his wrist. I curiously asked him one day, "Hey Javy why do you wear that thing?" He told me, "Huffy, I used to think so negatively. And it was dragging me down. So I put this rubber band on my wrist and every time I thought about something negative I would pull it back as hard as I could and snap my wrist with it. I would then immediately replace that thought with a happy memory, or thought." I took that advice and began wearing a rubber band around my wrist. After a month I had nearly broken skin.

You could also say I had been a control freak throughout my career, trying to control everything. I now realize that I had to let go. Trying to control things in my retirement was causing me even more anxiety and deepened my depression. Worrying about my future caused me anxiety because the uncertainty of it all drove me nuts. Thinking about my past as a baseball player depressed me because that was no longer my identity. I wasn't controlling anything! Anxiety and depression were controlling *me!* In order to move forward with my life, I had to rip off the rear view mirror, forget about Aubrey Huff the baseball player, and own my new identity as Aubrey Huff, the husband and father.

In the 1994 movie *The Shawshank Redemption,* Tim Robbins's character Andy Dufresne famously states: "Get busy living. Or get busy dying." I love that line because it perfectly sums up where I felt I was in my life. I had to get busy! I started working out again, if only to get me out of the house and around people again. I began to eat healthy. As a NPC fitness competitor and a certified personal trainer Baubi knows what she's doing when it comes to nutrition and fitness, so I leaned on her for inspiration. After a few months, the endorphins began to kick in and I started to feel hopeful again. I still took Xanax or turned to a few beers from time to time when I felt anxiety coming on, but I found myself needing the pills less and less. I was hell bent on ditching the Xanax forever! The beer however was a different story.

It's hard to fight the deep-ingrained white-trash DNA desire for an ice-cold Bud Light every now and then, but I had to completely ban alcohol for a while until I regained a sense of normalcy so I could kick the Xanax for good. I am happy to say that although I still enjoy the occasional drink today, alcohol no longer controls me.

With the booze out of my system, I now had to face my next demon. My ego! As a Major League Baseball player I sought validation from strangers. I would Google myself and read articles written about me by so-called journalists I had never even spoken to. I would pore over fan comments, most of them negative. Everything I was supposed to *not* do. As a human being I wanted to be liked, but at what cost? I had to drop my ego, get real, stop trying to impress and please others, and quit trying to be someone I wasn't.

But how was I going to lose my ego and still be confident, especially when confidence wasn't something I was born with? Confidence came easily as thousands of people screamed for me nightly. I felt invincible then, filled with a false sense of bravado. But that all took a kick to the nuts when I stopped taking Adderall. The end result was me walking away from the game, hating it.

I knew I couldn't be 'me' in my own strength. I had tried before and failed miserably. Then one day, a thought hit me like a slap to the face. *I don't hate baseball. I never did. It's me that I hate!*

How can I be confident when I hate myself? I still struggle with this today, but I now realize that being confident has absolutely nothing to do with me. Dropping my ego, letting go, and handing control over to God was the start. But I had to trust that Jesus was my only source of strength. This felt unnatural to say the least, because I had to have faith in something I could not hear, touch, or feel. When I did finally let go however, I was filled with a sense of peace, calm and fearlessness that is hard to describe. All I can say is that I know it didn't come from me. Because of this, I have the courage to write about my faith here, even though it is not popular or politically-correct.

It was now October 2015, a full year since I emerged from my closet, and months since my last Xanax. It had been rough sailing. I had lost many little battles, but finally felt like I was winning the war. I could see the light at the end of the tunnel, and it wasn't a Mack truck headed towards me.

Living in the present felt great. But that peace was fragile. I had spent a full year scared to let my thoughts wander to the past or the future, fighting the urge to even *think* about my next steps. The last thing I needed was another panic attack or bout of depression. But I couldn't live the rest of my life in a cocoon.

I saw a bright future for my wife and children. I loved being the best husband and father I could possibly be, but I needed to find something to be excited about when my feet hit the ground each morning. A positive end-goal to work towards every day.

I have to write a book. That thought had been nagging at me for a while now. I had no idea where writing would lead, or if it would even be any good. I just knew I had to start. It was a struggle, but as I stepped forward in faith, I found that I was finally excited to get out of bed each morning and grind away at a goal once again. Writing filled me with a sense of excitement I had not felt since I was a kid.

I am not writing this book for fame or money. I think I have already shared that those two things mean absolutely jack squat to me. I am doing it because I want to inspire others, and to finally break the vicious cycle that has dogged the Huff family for generations. I am convinced my father's alcoholism led to chronic depression. I know he left a path of destruction in his wake. His father, from what I have been told, was no different. I want all that to end with me, to break that destructive chain. To give my boys a shot at a future that is positive, healthy, and builds up those around them, instead of tearing them down. To be God-loving men who lead by example.

I am sure you realize by now that I am no biblical scholar. And again, please don't think I am preaching to you or that I'm rubbing this perfect life in your face. I'm not perfect. Far from it! I still have my bad days. Just ask Baubi!

I have absolutely no idea what the future holds for me beyond this simple dream, and that no longer frightens me, it actually fills me with excitement. But more importantly, I am excited knowing that one day I will be in heaven...in absolute paradise with my Lord and Savior Jesus Christ. I know now that my steps in this life are being guided by him, and that his plans far exceed anything I could ever hope or dream of. That faith was not easy to come by for me, but I now no longer worry about my future, or what I will be doing tomorrow or 50 years from now. My life is in his hands and that has filled me with an amazing feeling of freedom.

For years I thought that being a Christian meant being weak, and that Christians believe what they believe because they need something to lean on to help validate their fears. That day in the closet convinced me otherwise. Becoming a Christian actually made me stronger. But not until I realized that Christianity has absolutely nothing to do with religion. It's about developing a personal relationship with God. And like any relationship, that takes work.

I spent my whole career trying to be fearless, to keep all emotion bottled up. To never give my opponent any sign of weakness. I have had to unload mountains of guilt and resentment off my shoulders, desperately seeking relief with everything I could think of on this planet from medication, alcohol, drugs, yoga, therapy and meditation, to motivational books and videos. Nothing, not even the money and material possessions I acquired along my journey, was ever enough to fill that gaping hole in my heart.

Four years after hanging up my number 17, I can now proudly state that I finally have beaten my anxiety and depression. It no longer controls me. There is no longer a hole in my heart. The contentment, peace, and happiness I have found and enjoy almost every day now is indescribable.

I had risen to the greatest heights in my professional career. I had fallen to the greatest depths of depression and despair. And now, I had finally been redeemed.

But I'm just an average guy who has made massive mistakes in his life. I was lucky. A lot of guys never make it out alive. I got my life and family back. But it took my wife years to finally fully trust me again and let me back into her heart.

I struggled mightily with how to end this book. How do I summarize what finally lifted me out of that dark pit and gave me hope again in a politically correct way that doesn't simplify things too much, and doesn't offend anyone? I tried so many different ways to answer the question I am asked most, "How did I turn it all around?" It took me over a month to finally figure out what to write here.

Walking off the field victorious that final time in the 2012 World Series felt sad and unfulfilling. I would spend the next four years searching desperately, trying to find the real me. Trying to find my purpose in life. Trying to find *something* that would finally make me happy.

I finally found that something. I had searched high and low only to discover the answer was right under my nose the whole time. And for me it was so simple. Jesus. He is all I ever needed!

EPILOGUE

Late October 2016. Another gorgeous day in sunny San Diego, one straight out of the visitors and convention bureau's brochure. It sums up my mood perfectly. I stand next to Baubi at the kitchen counter as she labors, a beautiful smile on her face, cooking a healthy dinner for her three boys. Jayce and Jagger play happily on the living room floor.

I have finally found true happiness. Life can't be more perfect.